Pregnancy

How to Prepare Yourself to Be a Newborn Mama

(A Guide to Safe and Effective Workouts during Your First Pregnancy)

Kevin Jones

Published By **Andrew Zen**

Kevin Jones

All Rights Reserved

*Pregnancy: How to Prepare Yourself to Be a
Newborn Mama (A Guide to Safe and Effective
Workouts during Your First Pregnancy)*

ISBN 978-0-9948647-1-0

No part of this guidebook shall be reproduced in any form without permission in writing from the publisher except in the case of brief quotations embodied in critical articles or reviews.

Legal & Disclaimer

The information contained in this book is not designed to replace or take the place of any form of medicine or professional medical advice. The information in this book has been provided for educational & entertainment purposes only.

The information contained in this book has been compiled from sources deemed reliable, and it is accurate to the best of the Author's knowledge; however, the Author cannot guarantee its accuracy and validity and cannot be held liable for any errors or omissions. Changes are periodically made to this book. You must consult your doctor or get professional medical advice before using any of the suggested remedies, techniques, or information in this book.

Table Of Contents

Chapter 1: Preparing for Pregnancy

Things to consider prior to getting Expectant

Do you have a financial cushion? Are you in good health? Do you have prescriptions for drugs which may not be suitable for your growing child? Do you have a good partnership?

The financial security can be a benefit in the event that you want to grow your family. However, I wouldn't say it's an absolute requirement. If it appears that there's no way to start children if you need to be patient for financial stability, and you're mentally and physically capable of having a child then go for it. It's harder to rear children if you're on very little money, and you have nothing saved however it's not difficult. There may be times when you have give up the most expensive purchases and instead purchase products that don't come from a brand however it is possible to get it accomplished. Financial security guarantees that you won't need to cut back and save as often. However, the majority of families today have children while they're financially stable, only to go through a period of loss when they get laid off. If you're lucky there are family members who can help in times of need. If not lucky, there are federal programs that could assist you.

A further benefit is that you are well-nourished and healthy already. Weight is not a concern since there are lots of women who weigh a lot and healthy, however having a good weight prior to pregnancy is more attractive. It is possible to purchase outfits for your maternity if you're healthy and weight-wise, but it is more obvious that you're pregnant with your friends and family. But if you're suffering from diabetes, high blood pressure or another condition it could be an uneasy pregnancy than the majority. The majority of blood pressure medication are not suitable for use while pregnant. Certain medications can be, so consult your doctor prior to conception or immediately after it is discovered that you're expecting.

It's also crucial to evaluate your relationships. Are you a bit tense? Do you believe the birth of a child can make things more enjoyable than it already is? Do you have a significant other who is rude to or smack you or take advantage of you? If you've answered "yes" to these concerns this is not the ideal time to start planning the birth of a child. Be aware that you're adding the joy of a new baby to the table. If you don't feel safe, your child won't feel safe. One of the first questions that your child's caregiver or midwife may ask you at the time of your first visit. They are asking for the good of your child however they will also be asking for you. It is impossible to have the best pregnancy when you're constantly worried, distressed, or afraid.

How to Prepare for Pregnancy

In order to begin preparing for your pregnancy make appointments for consultations with several caregivers or midwives in order to select a caretaker who can be trusted and at ease with (see the steps to choose an OB/GYN or Midwife). Prenatal vitamins are taken every day as well as eat well-balanced meals and do some exercise. If you smoke and want to quit, stop. If you are a frequent drinker you should stop. If you take illicit substances, do not. If you're on medication prescribed by a doctor, speak with your physician to identify the right medication that's suitable for your growing infant. Start exercising, or keep exercise. Your health care provider will inform you whether or not you have to modify your workout schedule.

Ways to Increase Your Chances of Getting Pregnant

There are a variety of ways to boost your odds of becoming pregnant. If you do not want to create a career from it, simply get sex at a time you believe you'll be ovulating. If you do not be aware of when your ovulating There are a variety of ways to determine the moment you're ready to.

Ovulation predictor kits (OPKs) that are sold online and in your local supermarket will increase the chances of becoming pregnant. The majority of companies that offer pregnancy tests also produce OPKs. Certain OPKs are more difficult to interpret than others, therefore, you need to choose the most suitable one for you. What the OPK will do is identify the hormonal surge. Three phases are present to your cycle. They correspond to various hormones that are produced during certain periods. The first phase starts at the time you menstruate--the first day menstruation begins. This is known as the follicular stage. This is followed by the ovulatory stage. But, before the next phase begins the pituitary gland must released two hormones at the same time that are both stimulating the Follicle Hormone (FSH) as well as Luteinizing Hormone (LH). This is because of the increase in this hormone that OPKs detect. The increase in this hormone is crucial because it signals the follicle of your egg that it's time to let go and drop down through your fallopian tubes, and then insert its own (if it becomes fertilized) in the inner lining of your urinary tract. When this surge is identified, there is the opportunity to have a period of 24 to 36 hours within which your egg could become fertilized. The days following the surge, and also the day that you ovulate are the fertile days of your cycle. There are some women who do not experience an OPK-related surge despite actually being ovulated. The method involves that you pee on the stick (POAS) on certain days during your period. OPKs reveal the amount of surge (or the lack of it) by using a variety of methods. It is possible to purchase OPKs in digital format, such as a simple two-line OPK as well as a straightforward two-line OPK as well as an OPK with a happy face, or sad one.

Another method to increase the chances of having a baby is to chart your cycle. You can find and download charts to write your information on, or try a website like www.fertilityfriend.com to chart the cycle. The method varies from taking your temperature on a daily basis and examining your cervical mucus levels and the position of your cervix. It begins on the beginning of the menstrual cycle. When you wake up, you take your body's temperature at the basal level (you require the basal thermometer) prior to waking up, do some exercise and drink a glass of water. On the day prior to ovulation the temperature may drop a little. When you are ovulating, your temperature will increase and become greater than previous temperatures. When it does, you've already had your ovulation. Charting your body can help figure the time you usually ovulate within a few months after keeping track of your temperature every day. It is also possible to record information in the chart of the time you've had sexual sex, the way the cervical mucus (CM) appears and feels like, as well as the position of your cervical. The cervical mucus is shaped according to the hormones that are present in the body. Prior to ovulation it is when your CM changes from being thick and sticky into a liquid consistency just before the ovulation, it's an egg white consistency. Do not look at your CM following sex because during this time, it could be inaccurate. In order to check it correctly ensure that you have clean hands (fingernails are also clean). As you sit on the toilet or place one foot on the outside of the tub and then insert your fingers into the tub as deep as you are able to as you "scoop" out some mucus. The mucus you get from this is closest to the cervix, and thus, more pure. Egg white consistency is what you're looking for. The mucus which helps steer the sperm toward its goal. Cervix positions are difficult to locate if you're unintentionally "in tune" with your body. A lot of women cannot locate their cervix. It requires a lot of effort to discover exactly what is. If you do find it, you can feel the surface and take note of that, and also the location (high or low medium). If you are able to detect the opening, also record it (open or closed medium). In the days prior to and after ovulation your cervix should be large, wide, and soft. The hardness or softness of your cervix is generally related to the feeling of different facial areas. If it's hard and low, it'll appear like the top the tip of your nose. If it's large and soft, it'll look like the lips of your mouth. If it's extremely high, it can be difficult to identify. If you've not had children, your opening may be small and difficult to identify.

For those who don't want to spend money on OPKs each month, check their temperature on a daily basis, or check the CM or cervix. However, there is another option to monitor fertility. Fertility monitors can be a simple method of determining whether you're getting ready to become pregnant. Some require that you press an icon once per day, then inform the user when it's time to POAS.

The fertility monitors cost a lot and can be very useful. The first day you experience menstrual flow, you begin it in the morning. The on button is pressed the moment you awake, which gives you six hours for you to press the button. This is useful if the first day of the cycle falls on a weekend that's sleepy. When you press the button, it'll let you begin a new day when you push it for 3 minutes prior to or after the time you first push the button. When you begin your cycle, it will give you a POAS at approximately 6th day which continues until you have ovulated. If you're close to the time of ovulation it informs the woman that they are fertile. This is a pricey option, however If you're thinking about having multiple children this can help in getting pregnant quicker.

Having a Baby Is Literally Good for You

The birth of a child is a great way to make you feel happier. Once you have delivered your baby and especially when you're doing it without any medication, your body produces "love" hormones. It is like feeling satisfaction and joy. Your baby's eyes, take your baby's tiny hands, and feel a warm love for them. You'll be smiling more often when you see your baby develop and flourish. If you feed your child breastmilk then you're not just conserving money, and giving the child the one food which is made by your body in order to satisfy the demands of your baby as well as decreasing your risk of developing breast cancer.

When to Start Taking Prenatal Vitamins

Once you have decided to begin trying to conceive you should begin taking your vitamin supplements for pregnancy. If you've never seen an obstetrician, these vitamins can be bought over the counter. Aiming to use them for at least 2 months prior to conception could aid in ensuring that you're taking enough folic acids to lower the chance of a child born that has neural tube problems such as spina Bifida. Look for the prenatal vitamins that contain at minimum 800 mg of folate. The recommended dose for a not-pregnant woman is 400 mg (.40 mg) while for women who are pregnant, it's advised to consume 800-1000 mg (.80 or 1.0 mg) of Folic acid. A few of the prenatal vitamins you can buy over-the counter have 800 mg, however if you require more than that typically, you must take a prescription.

Chapter 2: Signs of Pregnancy

The Early Signs of Pregnancy

There are many indicators of pregnancy, and many may be identified as early when you begin to conceive. Here is a brief checklist of the signs will help you determine whether you're pregnant.

*Missed time

*Spotting in your regular period. Lighter and shorter than usual

Sore breasts

*Fatigue

*Bloating

*Period-like cramps

It is possible to spot it during your cycle (this could mean an implantation)

*Nausea

Strong sense of smell

*Darker areolas, nipples or darker

*Frequent urination

* Food urges

*Headaches

*Constipation

*Mood fluctuates

These are all indications of pregnancy, some of them can also be indicators of a coming menstrual cycle. There are two methods to know if you're actually pregnant.

Take a pregnancy test at home (HPT).

Be sure to find a test which detects minimal levels of Human gonadotropin chorionic (HcG) when you perform the test prior to when your period begins.

Ask your doctor to take a pregnancy test.

It is especially helpful when you've not had your period in a while, and HPTs do not indicate a positive.

Be aware that if there is no negative pregnancy test (either the blood test or HPT) You can request an ultrasound of the transvaginal area. Your caregiver can wait for some weeks to make certain that you didn't have an unnatural cycle. You must behave like you're expecting in this period. You should stop drinking, smoking as well as taking prescription drugs. make sure you take the vitamin supplements for prenatals.

When Do Signs of Pregnancy Typically Start?

Pregnancy signs may begin when you first begin to are able to conceive, however most of the time the signs don't show before you're six weeks old. Certain people do not show the symptoms. A woman I knew discovered that she was pregnant at was at 20 weeks of her pregnancy. Her cycles were unusual and did not believe there was something odd in not experiencing her period regularly. Also, she didn't have any of the pre-pregnancy symptoms. When she first felt the baby's movements when she realized she might be expecting. It is important not to depend on "typical" signs of pregnancy to reveal themselves. If you suspect you might be pregnant, consider taking the HPT.

HPTs cost starting at $1.00 and up to $15.00. It is the kind of test where you put a drop into a glass of urine. Another test is one that you use to urinate and display lines or indicators. Also, you can get digital HPTs that display the terms "Pregnant" and "Not Pregnant." There are times when you can purchase the test on the internet when you're having difficulty reading other tests.

How to Recognize Signs of Pregnancy

If you're attune to the body's signals, you could be able to detect indications of pregnancy very early. Women may feel the ovulating pain as a sharp ache in the upper or lower abdomen, which indicates that the egg has split from the ovary, and is now ready to drop. There may be a visible spots during the cycle, which could be an indication an egg that has been fertilized was in the uterine lining.

It is possible that sleeping on your stomach hurts the breasts. Breasts may become more fragile during the first trimester. However, they generally, they stop feeling tender prior to or in the second trimester.

The frequent need to urinate and nausea can also be seen early. While the fetus's size is smaller than tiny seeds at three or four weeks old the body is beginning to undergo transformations. It is an increase in HcG along with estrogen. The body is triggered to make more blood and that extra liquid needs to be flushed out. The common occurrence of nausea during pregnancy however the reason for it remains a mystery. Numerous doctors and nurses believe that the cause could be by an increase in HcG and estrogen. One reason that causes nausea might include an increase in your sense of smell. This can cause you to detect smells that you might not have been aware of before or become affected by smells common to you differently that you did when you weren't expecting. Whatever the reason, the most effective method to combat nausea is to take ginger. the ginger teas, lollipops drinks, and nutritional supplements are available in your the local grocery stores. Try eating crackers to ease nausea as well.

If crackers and ginger don't work well for you, or you're vomiting often and cannot eat food items, speak to your physician immediately. It is possible that you have Hyperemesis gravidarum. It is a rare pregnancy problem that can cause serious harm for the health of your baby. Hyperemesis is a condition which can persist throughout the pregnancy. It does not stop at the end of the first or second trimester like usual "morning" sickness does. Morning sickness is a possibility at any point, whether the morning, noon and at night, hyperemesis can occur during the daytime, no matter what you drink or eat. The condition can lead to the loss of water, weight as well as malnutrition.

Taking a Home Pregnancy Test and HCG Levels

A majority of tests for pregnancy at home can identify pregnancy up to five days prior to when your period is due. This test can be positive and negative. Eggs may be fertilized and implanted but they will be shed by the liner of the uterus. Women often experience "early miscarriages" after they use a sensitive HPT however, should they not have taken the HPT the women would be having their periods on time regardless and would not have known that they'd lost the child. Peeing on that stick can be extremely addicting. Every time you take a test, you're hopeful of a positive result, the dream of a child. A lot of chemical births (HcG and estrogen surges through the body but there's no sign of a foetus) are identified early by HPTs.

The highly sensitive HPTs are able to detect between 15mIU (mili International Units which is the amount of HcG within a amount of urine) of HcG, to up to 25mIU HcG. Some tests, like those that are less costly and also digital tests only provide positive results if the concentration of HcG present in your system is more than that; others are not able to register a positive until the amount of HcG within the system reaches 40 to 50mIU. Review the test's information tests available at the shop (or on the internet) to see how much HcG they can detect prior to purchasing one for a test that is early.

If you're having an early test there is no need to worry about which brand you choose because HcG numbers increase as you advance into your pregnancy. It is about the 12th week, when the numbers stop increasing. These numbers can be quite high, but they usually increase each day, but there are variations among women.

Choosing an OB/GYN or a Midwife

What you do with the baby of your choice is entirely your choice, however If you're looking for an unmedicated, natural pregnancies, then a midwife might be the right choice. Below are some of the things you should anticipate from both sides.

Obstetrician--

*Hospital delivery

*Medical intervention

Multiple tests, regular ultrasounds, monitoring of fetal growth during labor ultrasounds to determine the size of the baby, and pain treatment

Little one-on-one sessions in prenatal visits, typically around 10 or 15 minutes with your caretaker

*Current heartbeat at each appointment (sometimes carried out by the nurse prior to the caregiver is on the way)

• Ultrasound in 20 weeks

The mother is not able to see much of her mother during labor, up to the time of delivery

Laboring with your back giving birth from your stomach (some hospitals have different stances while others don't)

*Laboring in an in-tub (but not allowed to have water births)

It is not permitted to birth the baby in a natural way (Cesarean only)

Costs are based on your health insurance. A OB assisted pregnancy, even with no insurance, could run upwards of $9,000 (not comprising prenatal care such as ultrasounds, tests, or tests) And you'll be charged a separate amount for the baby.

Midwife--

Hospital delivery (in certain areas it is not possible to provide an in-hospital birth as per laws) and birthing centers delivery as well as home delivery.

* A few medical procedures

Testing can be done in any way you like and, in the event of a need and fetal monitoring is performed using an stethoscope. There is no medication for pain-management. These are natural, non-medicated births.

There is a lot of one-onone time is spent during appointments, typically 30-60 minutes depending on the amount you'd like to discuss.

*Heartbeats of the fetus at every appointment.

*Ultrasounds at 20 weeks (and only if medical conditions develop)

A near constant presence throughout the labor and birth

*Do whatever you like and delivering at the time/place that is most comfortable for you

*Water birth

*Will endeavor to give the most the breech positions

The cost of prenatal or delivery care for babies is typically less than $3500 from your the pocket (but there is a chance that you will get charged more for diagnostics or ultrasounds)

The reason for this is that OBs have been trained to treat pregnant women the same way as they treat other diseases. However, midwives are trained to handle pregnant women as a normal aspect of life. It doesn't mean that OBs aren't the wrong decision in any way. everything depends on your personal level of confidence. Certain women prefer OBs around, preferring to experience the hospital environment, but are scared of everything that could happen. Many women consider this decision restricting, and realize that the midwife is not going to allow them to deliver in their home or the hospital if there is a problem. If you're having difficulty laboring, make the decision that you would like an epidural or if the baby's experiencing distress, the midwife can call for an ambulance and get you transported to a hospital. The majority of caregivers won't allow delivery of a baby who is breech because they're not prepared to give birth to babies born breech. Midwives go through hours of instruction, part of which takes place in countries that are developing and are certified to perform most breech delivery positions.

For locating a service you can schedule multiple appointments with those you've picked. Make a list of your questions prepared. A few questions you can ask

What is the C-section percentage you have? (If you have a rate that is higher than ten percent, that might be a red alert for you.);

*How long am I permitted to stay pregnant prior to the induction? (The estimate of due dates can be described as it's an estimate. Pregnancies for first time mothers can go from 38 to 42 weeks. There are also cases of natural births occur around 42 weeks.)

Will you be accessible (not working or on holiday) in the vicinity that my due date is?

*Will you put in every effort to adhere to my plan of birth?

Which hospitals are permitted to give birth?

*How long do you have your prenatal sessions?

When are tests scheduled for certain dates or can I opt out of any?

There is a chance that you can identify additional questions to ask every OB and midwife. Another thing to be aware of is the level of attention that the midwife or OB gives to you when you're talking to them. Be attentive to particulars. Do they seem to be fidgety? Do they focus all their attention at you or appear as if they're trying to get somewhere? Are you comfortable being around them? If you're not comfortable around an individual who is dressed to the nines, you will not feel comfortable in a naked and unclothed person.

The First Prenatal Appointment: What to Expect

Prenatal appointments could be scheduled from seven to nine weeks, contingent on the history of your pregnancy and the level of stress your caregiver has. Once the pregnancy has been confirmed you should contact the caretaker or the midwife to schedule an appointment.

The initial appointment will generally be longer than other appointments, with the exception of that appointment when the midwife or caregiver tests to determine if you have Gestational Diabetes. The caretaker or midwife will establish your due date on the basis of the last cycle of your menstrual cycle, or after you've ovulated. The caregiver or midwife will inquire whether you've ever had pregnancies in the past and, if so been a victim of pregnancy, what happened? They'll want to know the results of previous surgeries. They will ask you for the medical information, which includes the history of your father and mother. They'll ask whether you drink, smoke or use medication (and the frequency of your use) as well as what there are any prescription or non-prescription medication you're using. Below are some of the tests that can be conducted.

The urine test can be used to determine for kidney infection, bladder disease and blood sugars (they could also utilize the test to conduct another screening for pregnancy);

A blood test (a total count of blood (CBC) that checks for problems with blood;

A HIV test (which is not required, however in the event that you've not had it do it);

*An examination for Rubella (they look for an immunity);

A test to determine if you are immune chicken pox.

*A hepatitis B test;

A blood type test is required to find out if you're Rh+, or Rh- (if it's your first baby, then the father needs to also be tested);

You can request genetic tests, where you and your partner are examined for markers of genetic origin for specific diseases.

A pelvic examination (your doctor will conduct an pap smear, if one is in the near future however, not when you've had it in the past two years. The doctor will put two fingers in the area to touch the cervix before he or the doctor will press onto your uterus in order to test to determine the size of your uterus actually is).

Placenta: How It Works

The placenta is an amazing innovation in the evolution of humankind. It helps eliminate waste, provide the infant with nutrients and also exchanges gasses through mothers blood. It begins to grow after the blastocyst (the egg that is still dividing into numerous cells) is implanted within the uterine wall. As the baby grows and the placenta expands. The flow of blood from mommy to baby is completely developed inside the placenta before the start of the second trimester. Umbilical cords connect the placenta to the baby and is essentially it is a dual-use road. Baby wastes are transferred through the umbilical cord into the placenta. During this process, the baby receives fresh nutrition. An unhealthy placenta can be described as an active placenta which can help your child develop and flourish.

Danger Signs in Early Pregnancy

The early stages of pregnancy are both thrilling and extremely stressful. It's when you develop the protective part of your brain. When you begin to realize how terrifying the process of introducing a baby into the world as well as the fear that an awful thing occurring to your child ever leaves you. There are some issues that could occur at the beginning of your pregnancy may be prevented if you seek medical attention immediately however, others can't. Your caregiver should be notified:

When you feel cramps that are severe. Don't think anything can be too minor--it could make the vital difference between living and dying;

If you see blood that is fresh (it is clear red and not brown as is an older blood type, and may contain clots and appear abundant or sporadic);

If you experience a fever or feel the chills (this could be a symptom of infection, and an high temperature may harm the embryo);

If you are feeling faint,

If you experience regular, painful urinations (this could be due to a bladder problem);

If you are suffering from an illness that causes fever, and you are vomiting.

If any of these signs are present, it's essential to see your caretaker immediately. If the caregiver you are seeing isn't accessible or it's at night, you can call the assistance number they have and/or go to the emergency department. If it's an illness, cold, or a placenta previa issue, your caregiver is able to assist in resolving the issue However, if the problem is previa placenta, the midwife won't assist you since you'll need the procedure of a C-section.

Chapter 3: Vitamins and Supplements

Choosing Your Pregnancy Supplements

Prenatal vitamins are an amalgamation of a variety of elements that are essential to ensure a healthy pregnancy. The choice of a supplement can be difficult since some might make your stomach upset, or induce nausea, especially if you're already expecting, or be deficient in the essential nutrients needed to sustain the health of your pregnancy. Discuss with your healthcare provider to select the appropriate supplements for you. If the supplements are causing difficulties, they could aid you in finding the right mix that works.

How Does Folic Acid Support a Healthy Pregnancy?

Folic acid is an essential ingredient of prenatal vitamin supplements. But, it is also able to be found in some food items.

Diets that are rich of folate (folic acid) will reduce the risk of birth defects which affect the brain such as spina Bifida. Certain foods that are rich in folate include

*Asparagus

*Spinach

*Avocado

*Peanuts

*Romaine lettuce

*Orange juice

This is just one of the food items which contain folate. There are numerous products that are packed with folate. If you consume your vitamin together with a balanced diet and exercising regularly, you're paving the way for a healthier pregnancies.

Why Is Iron Important?

Iron assists in moving blood throughout your body. It also makes hemoglobin, aids in strengthening your immune system and aids your child's brain grow.

From the time that you are born when you are born, your blood volume will begin rising. The blood volume increases by about 45% to the normal amount. Anemia is frequent in pregnant women who fail to have enough iron. It does not just affect the woman as well as the baby. The baby is able to store iron in the body that lasts for at least three months old.

There are a variety of foods that have iron in them and assist in keeping your levels of iron up. Some are

*Clams

* White beans

*Kidney beans

*Red meat

*Pumpkin seeds

There are many more but there are many more via research or speaking to your caregiver.

The benefits of fish Oil when pregnant

Certain prenatal vitamins contain DHA (a version that is derived from fish oils) included in these. DHA is believed to aid in the growth of the eye and brain in a fetus Certain studies have proven that taking 200 milligrams of DHA each day could increase the gestational time to at least 4 days. DHA is thought to lower the chance of

*Postpartum depression

* Cerebral palsy

*Gestational diabetes

*Preeclampsia

*Born prematurely

While it can help reduce this risk, it will guarantee that they'll disappear. In fact, taking DHA supplements could reduce the likelihood to develop the issues in your pregnancies, however different factors can raise your risk And sometimes, it's the case that it's just the way things go, regardless of what you do.

The Amount of Vitamins Needed for a Healthy Pregnancy

Keep in mind that these vitamins are simply supplements and it is important to eat food items that contain these essential nutrients. Since they're just supplements, it is possible to read the list of ingredients printed in the label on prenatal vitamins. You will find "Vitamin A 4,000 IU" and under the column marked the percentage of daily value as "50%." This signifies that the rest of 50% of your daily intake should come from the foods you eat.

If your doctor doesn't prescribe vitamin supplements for prenatal use and advises you to use supplements over-the-counter, look at the label on the bottle and search for supplements that contain the minimum amount of nutrients.

Vitamin A--4,000 IU (international units)

*Folic Acid--800 - 1,000 mcg

*Vitamin D--200-400 IU

*Calcium - 200-300 milligrams (mg)

*Vitamin C--85+ mcg

*Thiamin--1.4+ mg

*Riboflavin--1.4+ mg

*Vitamin B-6--2.6 mg

*Niacin (or B3)--18 mg

*Vitamin B12--4 mcg

*Vitamin E--15 mcg or 11 IU

*Zinc--11+ mg

*Iron--27-60 mg

If your supplements do not contain these requirements, then take additional supplements, or look for the brand that has these minimums.

Chapter 4: The Tests which can be performed during pregnancy

Types of Tests That Are Routinely Done at the Doctor's Office

Apart from the testing that you'll be given at your initial office visit There are additional tests your healthcare provider could carry out throughout the pregnancy.

The test you'll have to complete is called the AFP test, also known as the triple screen or quad screen. It is a test for neural tube disorders such as spina Bifida. It is sometimes employed to determine Downs Syndrome. The test is usually carried out between 15-17 weeks into pregnancy. This is a straightforward blood test that can be taken by the nurse's office as well as in a lab or a hospital. It is the most sensitive test within the specified time frame as well as if the dates differ by just a small amount, the result could be inaccurate. If the test comes back positive, you'll need take an additional and more thorough test. If the test is positive, it will are a cause for a level two ultrasound, or amniocentesis. Given the number of false positives depend on the beliefs you hold You can choose to not take this test and await an ultrasound scan at 20 weeks. If you'd like to continue to carry on the pregnancy regardless of what happens, the test will not be necessary and you are able to decide to decline it.

An additional test to be performed early is another test that is a precursor to the Nuchal Translucency screening test, through the process, they check to determine if you have Downs Syndrome. The screening is performed during the 11th to 14th week of pregnancy and can be done using ultrasound. An ultrasound will be able to determine the amount of nuchal fold. If the fold is large it is more likely to be at risk. If the test results are positive, the doctor may request for an amniocentesis, or an chorionic villus sample (CVS).

Amniocentesis may be a method to discover the presence of an chromosomal defect in the early stages of gestation. If it's done in the third trimester of pregnancy, it will be looking for baby's lung maturation (only when you're planning in labor or going to premature labor within 35 weeks). The procedure is carried out with the help of a doctor who inserts tiny needles through an abdomen to the incision of the uterus. Also, they perform an ultrasound simultaneously in order to guide to keep the needle from the baby or the placenta. The doctors collect a small amount of the amniotic fluid to examine for chromosomal abnormalities. The test is performed from as early as 11 weeks.

It is a CVS test is comparable to amniocentesis. However, it can be done at 8 weeks. Doctors use the ultrasound and needle and instead of entering by the stomach, doctors may also enter through the vagina close to the Uterus. The CVS test collects a tiny amount of villi in order to search for genetic problems. Results can indicate the normal birth or genetic disorder and may be used to determine the gender. The amniocentesis test and the CVS test are at risk of miscarriage. However, it is quite low ranging around 1 to 2 percent.

Other tests performed in the course of pregnancy include

*Gestational Diabetes tests typically occur between 24-28 weeks

*Ultrasounds

*Non-stress test (NST)--usually close to the due date, or if you are experiencing any

difficulties while pregnant. It is a test to determine whether your baby is stressed out or otherwise, typically done when you have passed the due date.

* Biophysical profile (BPP)--also scheduled for the day before due or when any health issues occur. This test tests the muscle tone as well as breathing patterns, as well as the amount of amniotic fluid. It is generally done if you're beyond the due date.

*Group B Streptococcus (GBS)--this test is performed to determine if you suffer from GBS in the vagina. The test is simple and a simple swab and is generally done before the due date. If the test is positive, your baby could develop it while he is out. Therefore, at the hospital, they'll administer intravenous antibiotics for 2 hours at least once. Your midwife might have alternative choices.

Ultrasounds: Why Are They Used and What Do They Serve to do?

Ultrasounds are used to direct needles during the CVS and amniocentesis. It is also used to conduct the BPP as well as to assist in determining the identify the time of birth (if you're not sure what time you had your baby) as well as track your child's development. An ultrasound at 20 weeks is the time when women usually learn the sex of their infant, but contrary to the popular opinion there is no reason why the ultrasound should be conducted. The ultrasound is used to measure the heart of the baby and ensure that it's developing properly, they take a look at the head, kidneys, bones and stomach. They examine the umbilical chord and observe the flow of blood to ensure it is functioning correctly. They monitor the heartbeat. The ultrasound technician can't give you the result. Results are passed to your doctor, who they interpret the results for you.

When Should I Decline Testing?

The test should be rescinded when you feel it is not necessary or you believe it is as medically injurious. Some tests should not be denied such as the GBS test, or the test for gestational diabetics. It is possible to decline all tests but if you choose to decline, your doctor could ask you to fill out the "against medical advice" (AMA) form to ensure their security.

Chapter 5: Pregnancy Diet

A Healthy Diet Is Important during Pregnancy

Dietary health is crucial when you are pregnant, because it will help the baby develop and keep your health as well. If you're not getting enough nutrition to yourself, then your baby is still getting the nutrients. Your baby's body is stripped of the nutrition it needs for growth. So, if you're lacking the necessary quantity of nutrition you require by your body, you're one of the people who is left without. Therefore, if you're one of those who consumes take-out meals on a regular routine, then a change in the way you eat is recommended if think of getting pregnant or already expecting.

What Are Some Healthy Pregnancy Diets?

There's an abundance of good pregnancy-friendly diets that can find on the internet or in books on pregnancy which is why I'm not going through each of them. Here are a few things to include in your diet when you're expecting or are thinking about becoming expecting.

*Legumes

It contains iron, protein and folate acid

*Meat (poultry and lean meat fish)

It is a source of protein as well as iron.

*Dairy (milk, yogurt, cheese, pudding)

It also contains protein, calcium vitamin B, vitamin D

*Fresh Fruit

Contains vitamin C

*Vegetables (sweet broccoli, corn asparagus (yeast extract)

Iron and folic acid are also present.

Do you remember the original FDA Food Pyramid? It was an all-purpose outfit that didn't take into account half people, since it was not designed for all. The new FDA food guidelines from www.choosemyplate.gov give you the ability to choose what's right for you. These guidelines are based upon the 2005 FDA Dietary guidelines. They include a picture of a table that will show you the proportions of each item ought to be included on your plate.

When you visit the site by the website, you will be able to enter your details into the questionnaire and receive an individual meal plan that is designed especially for your needs. In the case, for example, if you weigh around 120 pounds female, aged 28 years old, having less than 30 mins of physical activity per day the website will advise that you should consume a healthy diet.

6 ounces of grains

*2.5 cups of vegetable soup

*1.5 cup of fruits

Four cups of milk

Five grams of protein.

This is the amount of food you need to eat, if this is the case for your body makeup. This guide offers helpful suggestions for each food group and explains the foods you should look out for within that particular section. It is possible to create an account and keep track of your food intake along with your exercises, through the site. It is an excellent source for all. Start making use of it even before you are pregnant and begin to learn about eating in advance.

Choosing Healthy Snacks

A great way to choose a healthy snack is to follow the Food Guide Plate at www.choosemyplate.gov/food-groups.

This site will tell you how much these foods contribute to the daily allowance. If, for instance, you click on fruit after which an apple, you will see with a photo of an apple. And the apple will then tell the amount of cups of fruits it has.

Pick snacks that are healthy as well as avoid snack foods that are loaded with sugar and fat. The snacks you choose to eat should form included in your healthy, balanced eating plan. If you are beginning to follow a healthier diet, write down your plans before heading to the market. A way to stay away from eating fatty and sugary snack is to consume food before heading to the store. It will be apparent that you purchase lesser items off the list in the end, making it simpler to adhere to your shopping list.

Things to avoid when pregnant

Many women do not think about the items you shouldn't take in during your pregnancy. It is often difficult to stay away from certain foods since you might feel a need for them, however, recognizing that you're taking care of your baby and yourself can help to manage. If there's a particular one of these foods that you love throughout pregnancy, ask your spouse purchase the item when you're pregnant or the birth. This could be your celebration dinner! Here are some foods to stay clear of:

Deli meats and cold deli cuts can contain listeria that can result in miscarriages. They can also cross-contaminate the placenta and cause infection to the infant. If you simply must consume deli meat, heat it to a point where it's boiling and not cold.

Raw Meat: Raw meats are prone to many contaminants when pregnant, they is best kept away from.

Certain fish have mercury in them. Some have mercury contamination. Mercury levels are high within fish. Some contain the highest levels of mercury and others have low mercury levels. The caregiver you trust can provide specific guidelines on how much you can consume in a week, however the FDA recommends eating minimum 12 ounces of lower mercury fish each week. Some fish you should avoid (not the entire list) are sharks, Ahi tuna, and marlin. There is a six-ounce limit of tuna, sea bass and yellow tuna every month. There are 12 ounces of perch crawfish, catfish and clams, shrimps, tilapia as well as salmon per week. This list of options is expansive, so don't think as if you're limited to a certain amount if you enjoy seafood.

*Smoked and raw seafood - they contain many toxins that could affect your health when you are pregnant and must be completely avoided. That means you should avoid raw oysters or other sushi, and even seafood cooked is at risk of being affected by contamination. It is common to cook the sushi with the same surface.

There is an increased risk of salmonella contamination in eggs, it is advised to steer clear of any food which contain eggs that are raw for example: Caesar salad dressings, mayonnaise, custards made from scratch, or eggs cooked in a hurry.

Soft cheeses are imported and include listeria. They include Brie, Roquefort, Feta and Mexican qusoblanco.

Be sure to wash your produce, particularly when you are doing yourself gardening. There is a risk that soil may contain Toxoplasmosis thanks to neighbors' cats. It could be a source of a rare blood borne infection.

Healthy Pregnancy Eating Habits

Do not let the old adage, "I'm eating for two now, I can eat what I want," become your mantra when you're pregnant. This could lead to eating too much as well as eating plenty of food that isn't healthy, and even gaining weight. Do not think of the new way of eating as a way to lose weight, or a diet. It's more of a lifestyle change There's nothing which says that you cannot continue living that way after you've had your child. Women who are pregnant require between 2200 and 1500 calories per day that is higher than the average amount needed by pregnant women. This isn't an enormous distinction, however this is why some women fall into the trap of eating too much. An average, healthy woman is eating between 1600 and 2200 calories per each day. Look at the back of your products for serving sizes of food and the number of calories per portion. Be sure to check the amount of sodium and fat each portion has. If you notice that the amounts are higher than you expected the reason is that it's too processed. You can try using freshly prepared ingredients to create identical products. Add a bit more time in your daily schedule to cook your meals and you'll be amazed by the result.

How to Control Pregnancy Junk Food Cravings

In the battle to control your cravings for junk food, it isn't easy. Make sure to keep this food part from your daily diet, as you might be tempted to binge and eat way too much. It is better to buy smaller amounts (1 portion size) to use at a time when you will most likely not be able to replace for something other than this one. Some substitutions can help you get through until the next time you are craving something. As an example, instead of eating chips made from potato Try pretzels or popcorn with a low fat content. It is possible to substitute an granola bar that is low in fat to make a candy bar, or raisins or dried fruits to make sweet treats that are crunchy. The trail mix (without chocolate) could be an excellent alternative. As an alternative to ice cream go for pudding or yogurt. If you're looking for soda, try drinking the juice of a fruit. If bubbles are what you want, get seltzer water that you can put into your juice. Try to stay away from junk food however, don't be too hard on yourself when you indulge at times.

How Much Water Do You Need?

Drinking water can help keep you satisfied. Additionally, it aids in transporting essential nutrients to the body. It is recommended to consume at least eight

8-ounce glasses per daily, however it does not need to be water. It is possible to drink beverages like milk, juice, or beverages that have caffeine in them or have been not decaffeinated. But, it is important to restrict your intake of caffeine. Drink whenever you're thirsty or when you are doing light activities. The effects of dehydration could trigger labor early If you begin to contract at an early time (and it's not uncomfortable) take a drink and lay on your back. If your ankles, legs or hands become swollen, take more fluids. Water isn't what keeps you hydrated, and drinking more water can aid in reducing swelling.

Chapter 6: Fitness in Pregnancy

How Does Fitness Help You Have a Healthy Pregnancy?

Being fit or healthy during pregnancy could assist in the fight against the effects of high blood pressure, aches and pains. It can also reduce the chance of developing gestational diabetes or undergoing an emergency C-section.

Tips for Healthy Exercise during Pregnancy

If you exercise prior to your pregnancy, keep exercising regularly, typically until you notice it difficult or following the recommendation of your doctor. Be sure to drink plenty of water while you exercise. If you feel discomfort or cramps during exercise, you should stop. Ask your doctor what exercises are safe for you and those that aren't. If you're not active or sedentary it is possible to start taking a walk every day. Walking is safe from 30 to

60 minutes per day. It isn't necessary to do it all simultaneously or to be a vigorous walk.

How Pregnancy Yoga Helps You Keep Fit and Healthy

Yoga can help you remain fit throughout pregnancy, it also helps in the birth of your child. Yoga makes your body agile, allowing the use of a range of positions throughout labor. It helps you stay at peace and helps reduce stress. It can help enhance your posture, which could help back pain that are caused by pregnancy. This can help improve your pelvic floor following pregnancy it will strengthen your abdominal muscles that are stretched through pregnancy.

What is a Healthy Pregnancy Weight Gain?

The weight gain during pregnancy is different from woman to. An average gain of 30 pounds. However, it is possible to be quite different. The caregiver keeps an eye on the weight you are carrying and will ensure you're within the limits. If you're obese and you are losing weight, it's possible that you will shed weight, and your caregiver isn't going to be concerned except if there isn't enough food.

The typical gain is between 1 and 4 pounds throughout the first three months. Then, you'll add up to 2-4 pounds every month for the following two trimesters. It is possible the weight gain increases towards the close of your cycle.

What to do to Avoid Gaining too much weight during pregnancy

In order to avoid gaining excessive weight, adhere to a balanced and healthy diet, as well as exercise frequently. If you're at the couch, you will not have the time to work out yet, however you are able to consume a healthy diet. Beware of snacking on snacks, chocolate, or soda pop. Don't forget that dessert doesn't have to accompany every meal.

Chapter 7: Sex during Pregnancy

What is the best way to have sexual relations while pregnant

It is possible to have sexual sex however you'd like in pregnancy particularly if you are having a low-risk, uncomplicated pregnancy. Most of the times, the only thing stopping you from performing something is your personal preference. There is no reason not using sex toys throughout pregnancy. Just be careful not to penetrate them too deeply and clean them regularly so that you don't get infection. Sexual sex for oral purposes isn't completely out of the question However, at the time of termination you and your partner might be uncomfortable down in the midst of all the fluids that your body produces. Keep in mind that sex won't harm the baby in any way. If it's not a good idea for you or your baby, your caretaker will notify you.

A few of the most comfortable position for sexual intimacy during pregnancy is women-on-top, side-to-side and intercourse with your back. The more advanced you get during this pregnancy stage, the more relaxed certain positions can be. You are free to try different positions and let your spouse be aware of any discomfort or are in discomfort. If you're not comfortable sexually, you can remain close to your spouse. It is possible to mutually masturbate or touch, hug and kiss one another. Be careful not to let your aversion hinder your love affair. There's a chance that the occasional relationship can actually enhance your bond.

What are the benefits of a Sexual Pregnancy?

There are a lot of benefits sexual intimacy with your partner may bring for as long as you're married to one another and you do not have a concern about developing sexually transmitted infections. There are many benefits the fact that it

The baby is relaxed by the motion of rocking and gentle squeezes of your uterus while your gasm gently rock the baby back to sleep.

Induces labor when your body's already gearing toward labor. Although this has not been proven through any studies conducted by scientists, numerous caregivers recommend that it is the case.

It helps you connect with your spouse--sex may assist you in becoming closer to your spouse through the often difficult times of your relationship.

Preparing the pelvic floor in preparation for labor. Sex helps tone the muscles that you'll utilize when it's time to welcome baby;

Feels wonderful - your body is changing as it goes through changes, and you'll experience new and amazing sensations you've probably have never felt prior to.

Oral sex may also induce the process of labor. Recent research has shown that the prostaglandins in semen help initiate labor faster if semen is consumed. It's not for everyone, however!

When is Sex Allowed and When Is It Not Allowed?

There are many reasons people are told not to go out. Many of them are based about pregnancy related issues. The likelihood is that sexual activity could be banned by your primary family doctor in the event of a pregnancy-related issue.

If you have been in preterm labor

You have a placenta previa

*Your water breaks are at the end of every day,

If you have a past pattern of miscarriages

You have an unfit cervical cervix.

You experience heavy bleeding.

Keep in mind that if your doctor states you can't have sexual relations that means there are no orgasms, either.

Chapter 8: Healthy Sleeping in Pregnancy

Sleep during Pregnancy

Being able to fall asleep while pregnant particularly towards the last part of your pregnancy can be difficult. However, it's not difficult. In your first trimester, you shouldn't be having any issues sleeping, and you will probably sleep more frequently.

What are the best sleeping positions for Pregnant Women?

It is recommended to sleep on your left side. is the ideal position to pregnant women, particularly toward the third trimester. It may be much more relaxing to rest your body on pillows in case you're experiencing burning sensations in your stomach. Do not sleep on your back as it places stress on the Aorta as well as the Vena Cava that can reduce the flow of blood for your body as well as your infant.

Additionally, it increases your risk of developing hemorrhoids, heartburn and lower blood pressure.

You'll sleep better throughout Pregnancy

Here are some tips to help you get more restful sleep during the course of pregnancy.

Stop drinking caffeine-rich drinks that are not recommended in any case. If you do have to consume the drinks, make sure to avoid drinking them prior to bedtime.

Do not consume fluids prior to the time you go to bed or consume a large dinner prior to going to bed.

Create a schedule for getting up and sleeping in the same order each evening.

Take a bath (not overly hot) in the evening before going to bed. Relax.

Get up, read, or play music or something that will distract you from the fact that it is impossible to go to sleep when you're in a trance and are getting frustrated.

Buy a body pillow ease pain throughout the evening. There are special "pregnancy" pillows that you could purchase to accommodate the body of a pregnant woman.

Chapter 9: Oral Care during Pregnancy

How to Take Care of your teeth during pregnancy

Cleanse your teeth in the same way as you do throughout pregnancy, and make sure you floss your teeth regularly. As you grow as a new baby, you will require more calcium. If you're not getting sufficient calcium, your body is able to take it out of the bones and teeth. Consult your dentist within your first trimester to get a dental cleaning in case you didn't have one already. make sure that any tooth decay is taken care promptly.

Why Are Your Gums Sensitive During Pregnancy?

When you are pregnant the body undergoes numerous changes due to hormones. Progesterone levels that are higher than normal levels as well as the elevated blood levels can cause the gums more sensitive throughout the course of pregnancy. If your gums are swelling they store the bacteria that cause cavities, and can cause irritation to gums, causing them to increase in size. A lot of pregnant women suffer from tooth decay near the gum line because of this.

Bleeding Gums during Pregnancy

As your gums become more fragile, you'll see some pinkish spots in your basin when you brush and brush your teeth. It's due to hormones of pregnancy as well as your elevated blood pressure. This is an usual pregnant symptom, also known as pregnancies gingivitis. The reason why you're experiencing greater bleeding from your gums in comparison to normal like I mentioned is that hormonal changes cause your gums to become more prone to bacteria that can cause gingivitis and plaque. But don't fret, this does not mean that you're more likely to developing gingivitis when your birth is finished. Go to the dentist frequently to get your teeth cleaned and floss and brush every day at least two times.

How Cavities Can Affect Your Pregnancy

However, women who normally don't develop cavities could find that their teeth are getting more being pregnant. As your gums expand they also trap food particles and bacteria. This not just causes bleeding, and also leads to cavities along your gumline. The ideal time to have dental treatment is in the second trimester. In the first trimester your fetus begins to develop organs, and it's the most vulnerable because it's not dependent completely on the placenta until it is in the second trimester. Due to this, it's best not to the exposure of your baby to harmful radiations and chemicals. Letting your back rest during long periods isn't good for your back in the third trimester. It is recommended to hold off until after birth to have any tooth fixed. However, if it's an emergency situation, Novocain and some antibiotics can be used safely while pregnant. A majority of dentists do not request an entire set of x-rays during pregnancy and if the dental issue is in a bad state the dentist may take x-rays of that particular tooth.

However, can gum and tooth problems affect the fertility of the baby? Yes it is possible. In the case of gum disease, it can result in preterm births and weight loss at birth. Additionally, women with dental cavities during pregnancy have babies with higher risk of develop cavities prior to reaching the age of 5.

Chapter 10: Work Meets Pregnancy

Work during pregnancy what to do and not do

There's no reason to believe that women shouldn't work in the event of becoming pregnant. If you're not instructed to stop your work by your doctor and you are able to continue working until you are in labor.

Beware of scents that could trigger vomiting or nausea.

Do snack frequently and keep crackers or Melba toast in your bag to ease nausea.

Keep a bottle of ginger ale or tea on hand.

Do drink plenty of fluids. Keep drinking bottles or a personal water container that is filled with water and on hand throughout the day.

Do not work till you are done.

Do take breaks.

Do stand up and walk around when you tend to sit, or sit in a comfortable position and unwind if your job requires lots of standing.

Do not hide the fact that you are pregnant from your boss. It is important to let them know that you're pregnant and will need to take a break. In the event that they do not, they might believe that you're not working!

What Can You Do to Promote a Healthy Pregnancy at Work?

If you are working in a place that is risky you should mention it to the person who supervises you. There may be a need to change the work you perform could cause harm for a baby growing. Certain jobs can lead to difficulties during pregnancy, specifically in the event that you're susceptible to premature labor. In particular, if you have to work with hazardous chemicals, huge machinery, cold and extreme environments and excessive noise it is important to determine whether you are able to be relocated into a more secure position after the birth. Once you've talked to your caretaker, talk to your manager about any potential issues.

Relax often and be careful not to go overboard. If you are overwhelmed you should take a moment to relax. Locate a calm place in which to relax until you're more relaxed. Speak to the person(s) who cause anxiety, or talk to someone else like a coworker or a friend. Discussing your concerns could help reduce the stress that is causing them.

How Does the Stress Level at Your Job Affect a Healthy Pregnancy?

Stress of any kind can influence pregnancy, however work-related stress usually ranks on the highest of chart. Stress triggers chemicals (cortisol) signals throughout the body, and then into the placenta. Cortisol may cross the placenta. However, the impact of cortisol on a pregnant fetus over a long period is not fully understood. The long-term cortisol exposure for adults could result in depressive, fatigue as well as high blood pressure. This can affect your pregnancy, creating a greater challenge for you to get work done, or to focus on anything else or anything, and elevated blood pressure may cause preeclampsia. Keep in mind that you're not just growing and taking care of a child and your baby, you need to begin taking care of your well-being. Reduce your stress at work by reducing anxiety by

*Exercising regularly

Prenatal yoga classes are a great way to prepare for birth.

Learning relaxation techniques to help you relax during pregnancy.

Relaxing and taking a break whenever the levels of stress get way too high

*Walking

Breathing in thoroughly (breathe in slow through your nose until the number five Exhale slowly and then exhale through your mouth until you reach the number of eight. Repeat.)

• Cuddling with your spouse, pet

Massages for pregnant women

Relaxing music

Thinking positively

It is possible to control the level of stress that you feel both at work and home. The most difficult part is letting release the tension you are causing because of your work instead of wallowing and wailing.

Chapter 11: Common Pregnancy Ailments
Yeast Infection during Pregnancy

The yeast lives in moist, warm and dark, sweet places. It flourishes the most in pregnancy due to the additional wetness that pregnancy hormones produce, as well as the increased amount in sugar content of the discharge. It is possible that you will notice increased discharge during your time pregnant. If the discharge is odorous or is odorous to it, often accompanied by itching, it could be due to a yeast infection. Be wary of self-diagnosis and instead report the issue to your doctor. It's a quick simple test, and it could indicate a vaginal infection such as Bacterial Vaginosis that may result in preterm pregnancy. The antibiotic Diflucan that is typically given to women who are not pregnant, hasn't been confirmed in the presence of pregnant women. Instead, your doctor may prescribe or prescribe the use of an antibacterial cream or suppository to apply for a period of 7 - 14 days.

Pregnancy Constipation: Are Stool Softeners Safe?

Constipation is an atypical consequence of being pregnant. There are several over-the-counter stool softeners suitable for use when pregnant (don't use laxatives while pregnant) However, talk with your doctor for advice on what's most suitable for your needs. If you're looking to stay away from taking medication, there are several alternative options that are natural to stool softeners.

* Drink more fluids

*Drink the juice of a prune

Eat foods that are high in fiber.

*Eat apples, raisins as well as bananas and rhubarb.

How to Maintain a Healthy pregnancy with hypertension

It is possible to have normal blood pressure if you're not pregnant, but when your healthcare provider notices that your blood pressure is slightly higher than usual. The blood pressure can be classified as high when it is 140/90+. Normal readings are about 130/70. If you're experiencing high blood pressure readings, your doctor is likely to begin paying attentively to the reading. The high blood pressure that occurs during pregnancy may result in

If the blood pressure of your excessive, your doctor could choose to perform a preterm delivery in order to stop any serious health issues to you or your newborn.

A decrease in blood flow to the placenta - the placenta is the vital source for your child. The lower blood flow indicates the baby doesn't get adequate nutrients or oxygen, that could lead to IUGR (inter Uterine Growth Retardation) also known as SGA (small to gestational age) that may result in premature birth.

This can create problems for the infant as well as the mother. It's considered as a serious condition for babies, because the baby is deprived of nutrition and oxygen. The condition could cause the need for a C-section.

This disorder typically manifests at the time of delivery, however, it can occur earlier or even post-delivery. The condition can be life-threatening and cause early induction or even a C-section.

If you're already hypertensive and you are taking medications prior to conception, talk with your physician about the medications you are taking and be certain they're safe for you for you to use during pregnancy. If you've been diagnosed with hypertension while pregnant, your healthcare provider might prescribe medications to treat the condition. Certain blood pressure medicines are considered to be safe for pregnant women however, most medicines can cross the placenta, and pose risks for the child, the caregiver determines whether to give the medication based depending on the risk or rewards. If the potential risk associated with the drug is greater than the benefit and the medication is not prescribed, your doctor will decide not to prescribing the drug.

Lower your blood pressure by working out and eating a healthy diet. Consider diets that call on natural ingredients. Check out documentaries like Forks over Knives to learn what eating healthy can do to improve your health as well as reduce your dependence on medication.

What can you do to Prevent Stretch Marks throughout Pregnancy

As your body expands rapidly the skin expands in order to match the growth of your body. In pregnancy, the skin expands extremely quickly. The next day, you awake and then you appear to be pregnant. If your skin is stretched quickly, elastin could be damaged, causing stretch marks. There's a myriad of creams and ointments available on shelves that promise they will prevent stretch marks. However, the reality is that there's no way to stop stretch marks. The cause of stretch marks has something to do more with your genetic make-up and less using the creams or the ointments that you put on your belly. If your mom made it through pregnancy with no stretch marks most likely you don't be either, or only a small.

Creams and ointments won't eliminate stretch marks, they may reduce those appearances of the stretch mark and this is when the products are useful. Find pure creams and ointments however, because a large portion of the commercial ones contain chemicals that could be hazardous and aren't evaluated for their safety when pregnant. Additionally, if you suffer from delicate skin, these products could cause a lot of trouble and make you sleepless at night. The most effective way to avoid or reduce the appearance that stretch marks appear is reduce the stress level, boost fluid intake to keep skin hydrated using natural creams or oils (try Vitamin E) and eat nutritious food items, and monitor your weight increase. In the end, when you do develop stretch marks, do not allow them to bother you. They're a sign of motherhood, and only stunning women are proud to wear them. They also tend to fade from being angry and red anger as time goes past, and transform to soft silvery lines that are only visible in specific lighting.

What can help reduce swelling in feet during pregnancy?

There are many options to ease and reduce swelling of feet in pregnancy. There are some suggestions to test.

Drink more water! Fluid retention is one of the main causes for swelling of feet, drinking a lot more fluids can reduce swelling. It is an attempt for the body to store the water that you're not drinking enough.

Put your feet up.

Stay off the floor for hours in a row.

Wear shoes that are comfortable. It is moment to eliminate those high heels. In addition, feet alter sizes during pregnancy.

Be sure to keep track of during your during your pregnancy.

*Give your feet and legs a bath with Epsom salts.

Ask your companion to provide you with the massage of your feet to ease the pain.

Strategies to Reduce pressure on the Pelvic Area during the Final Trimester

When you get closer to the due date, you might feel more pressure on the pelvic floor. At times, it's like your baby's head is in the middle, waiting to pop out. However, it's not an enjoyable sensation. When you are progressing through your pregnancy, your baby begins to adjust its body to get ready for birth. It can be uncomfortable, and there are some ways to alleviate that discomfort but the only way to get rid of the discomfort is to have a baby.

*Lie down on your left

Use a belly band, or sling. It helps to keep your uterus in place.

*Change position

*Take a relaxing bath

Place yourself in a seated position on your knees and place your head in between your hands, keeping your torso at 20 minutes in intervals.

The last one can alleviate pressure and also help position the baby better, loosen the pelvic floor and ease back discomfort.

Chapter 12: Complications That Can Occur

What is Gestational Diabetes?

Although you've not had diabetes in the past, consume a balanced diet and don't have any excess weight and fit, you could be diagnosed as being gestational diabetic. There's not a lot of reason for this to happen however, in certain pregnancies it is the case that the body isn't in a position to make sufficient insulin to regulate your blood sugar. When you're pregnant, and your blood sugars rise over normal levels, you'll be asked to test the blood sugar level four every day. You may also sometimes you will be asked to record your meals consumption. If you're unable to reduce your level through diet alone and you are prescribed insulin. One reason for keeping an eye on for the signs of gestational diabetes is because it may have detrimental consequences for the infant.

Gestational diabetes may make your baby's blood sugar levels. This increases the pancreas of your baby's the levels of insulin. It also produces more energy, and converts that energy into fat. This leads to macrosomia (a obese baby). Macrosomia can:

*Leads to weight issues in the future.

Increases the likelihood of a child being diagnosed with Type 2 diabetes that develops in adults.

The shoulder dystocia can be caused by birth

The breathing difficulties in newborns can be caused by a variety of factors.

• Low blood sugar levels at time of

The test of blood glucose levels usually takes place between the 24-28th week, based on the advice of your physician. The mother usually suffers when the baby's body has formed (it includes all of its digits and appears as a baby) however, before they've fully increased in weight or size. The most effective way to prevent gestational diabetes, or manage the condition once it's been identified is to adhere to a nutritious diet that is low in sugars as well as processed food items.

What is Fetal Demise?

Fetal demise is a medical term used to describe a child that died within the infancy. Pregnancies that are healthy can change to the worst. Baby that was running around and playing in the tummy of your child suddenly ceases to move, or, in some cases, there's no reason to believe or explanation of the child's loss. If you've experienced this then the most effective thing you can discuss your emotions with your partner or join with other mothers who've experienced the loss of a child, or be part of a group that offers support to women who've experienced the loss. Allow yourself to mourn. The loss of a child during any time of pregnancy is difficult for each of you. It may seem as if he's suffering exactly the way you do however, he's. Each person grieves each way in their own manner, so it's important that they have enough time for grieving.

There's nothing you can do to help you prepare for the worst regardless of the fact that you know the baby is an unborn baby, you believe that perhaps your doctors are wrong and the baby may weep. The baby's heart will beat in your palm when you place its tiny body in your fingers. It'll turn its eyes to look at your face. This isn't always the scenario. If this happens to you this is among the most difficult things that anyone could bear. Be aware that the risk that your fetus will die affect your pregnancy. However, realize that this is a possibility which can occur. If this does occur do not blame yourself for it. You shouldn't believe that there was some kind of sign in some place, that you might have noticed if you'd paid to pay attention. This isn't the norm all the time.

Try doing counts of kicks. You can count the number kicks your child is making in an hour. If the baby kicks at a rate of less than 10 times one hour, contact your physician. If you're experiencing contractions and are in late-mid-pregnancy, consult your physician. If you smoke, or take substances, you should stop. Using these items can increase the chance of stillbirth. Let your doctor know.

When you have a still-born child, your doctor will conduct tests to see whether they are able to determine what caused the death of your baby. Blood tests are conducted to determine if there are genetic issues. They'll ask you to would like an autopsy. They might even request some kind of test for drugs. Results can help determine the cause of your child's death and prevent future deaths from occurring later on. Sometimes, however, no cause could be identified. The baby may have died or stopped growing, and there is no explanation as to what caused it. Sometime, I believe it's the hardest aspect - not knowing the reason. It's possible to rant and shout and get angry and rage, but there is nothing to point it at. If you could tell it was due to a specific factor, or a specific factor, then you'd know who you were to take the blame for.

When you've lost a child, you're at a more risk of getting another. It's entirely your decision what date you're likely to attempt a second time. The doctor who is treating you will likely advise you to wait for at least 3 months prior to making another attempt, in order to not just give your body the time it needs to heal but also allow your heart to recover.

Chances of being stillborn baby are greater the mother is not present.

If you are 35 or older, then you're eligible.

You are overweight

You smoke cigarettes or drink alcohol

You take a prescription drug

*You've had previous stillbirths

*You've taken pain medications during pregnancy

You have high blood pressure.

If you have liver disease, it is likely that you will

You have a family background of blood clots

If you have a multiple pregnancy (more than one child)

*You are African-American

The baby you have isn't growing.

You've been involved injured in an accident, fell or suffered physical abuse

Inform your doctor that you're suffering from one or more of the above risk factors.

What is Preeclampsia?

Preeclampsia usually begins at around the 20th week. The condition affects the placenta of the infant as well as the mother's kidneys. It usually manifests as an abrupt change in blood pressure. It is a sign that your blood pressure is elevated compared to normal. When seizures begin and then progress to Eclampsia and is among major causes for mother-to-child deaths within the United States. There's no reason for it. for preeclampsia, and the sole way to treat it is to deliver the infant. If the preeclampsia you are suffering from is serious or it progresses to fully-blown Eclampsia and your doctor decides to initiate or conduct C-section even when you're not close to the due date. The reason for this is to protect the life of you, and as well to ensure the life of the baby should it be it is possible. Preeclampsia can

Prevent your baby's placenta isn't supplying the baby with nutrients via the bloodstream. They don't get enough nutrients;

The placenta is calcified by the placenta;

*Diseases that can lead to early birth

*Turn into Eclampsia and could cause seizures as well as coma or death.

What Are the Signs of Preeclampsia?

There are indicators that the doctor will be looking at to see whether you suffer from preeclampsia. The doctor or caregiver will search for the following signs of preeclampsia

*High blood pressure

*Protein found in the urine

Extremities swelling that is rapid

* Rapid weight gain

*Dizziness

*Seeing spots

*Faintness

*Nausea and vomiting

*Humanitis severe

If you are suffering from these symptoms the doctor will typically recommend a complete or part-time bed rest. If the situation is not ideal, your caretaker will require you to stay at the hospital to be under surveillance. This gives your baby the chance to grow in the event that your health deteriorates, your baby will have a better chance of survival if you must deliver the baby early. Your doctor might prescribe medication to treat the illness, in the event that you're getting close to the due date for delivery, you might choose to induce.

Other Complications to Watch For

Unfortunately, the pregnancy process isn't a wonderful experience for all women, and there are complications that do occur. It's impossible to prevent everything that's bad from occurring and nothing is possible to predict. A few of the issues that could occur during the normal and healthy pregnancy are preterm labor the abruption of the placenta, gallstones, the presence of amniotic fluid in low levels, and previa placenta.

Preterm labor refers to labor that occurs prior to the 37th week of the pregnancy. If you begin experiencing frequent contractions prior to 37 weeks pregnant and they're making the cervix to expand and erupt, you could be having preterm labor. It is possible that you are in premature labor in the following situations:

*You experience four or more contractions per hour or you are suffering from painful like cramps that resemble a period.

Your discharge may change, becoming more liquid mucousy, bloody, or mucousy

There is pressure on the pelvic region that is higher than usual

It is a numb or a pulsating backache.

*You're bleeding.

* Your water stops working

If you are experiencing one of these signs contact your doctor promptly or visit the closest emergency room.

Preterm labor is usually reduced in the hospital as well as many women that go through preterm labor are able to give birth within the 37th week gestation.

Placental abruption occurs when the placenta begins to break away from the uterine wall prior to when you give birth to your baby. It could be hazardous for the mother as well as the child. Signs include:

*Vaginal bleeding that can occur fast, or progress gradually, and can range from in the range of pink or deep red

Abdominal pain, uterine tenderness,

*Back pain,

Rapid contractions, with no time between.

If you are experiencing one of these signs, contact your doctor immediately. It's impossible to repair the placenta after it has been ripped out of the uterine wall. However, given the proper care, you may be able to deliver a healthy child. The caregiver will likely have you hospitalized for careful surveillance, and in certain instances, they'll give the baby steroids in order to make your baby's lung develop. If bleeding ceases and your child is in good health Your caregiver could allow you to in your home. Bed rest is intended to keep your placenta safe from further tearing, so it's crucial to adhere to the directions of your caretaker. If you're near the time of delivery, your caretaker may choose to birth the child, whether by C-section or through induction dependent on the severity of the suddenion.

Gallstones from inside your gallbladder. They can create pain if they break away out of your gallbladder. They can end up stuck in their journey out. They may obstruct your liver, causing an overflow of bile into the stomach. It is true that women are more susceptible to developing gallstones in pregnancy. Gallstone symptoms include:

There is severe pain on the upper portion of your abdomen, or between the shoulder blades (it will not be the same for all people)

Indigestion and nausea (worse than the normal)

*Neon, dark, or orange yellow urine, or light-colored stool

Eyes' skin, white or even the eyes' becoming yellow

The form of care that you get for gallstones is contingent on how serious the gallstones in your body are (the caretaker can arrange an ultrasound scan to determine what the extent of the problem) and also how far the pregnancy process is. Your doctor may recommend medication and pain pills to treat gallstones. If you're in the second trimester they could choose to eliminate the gallbladder since surgery is the most secure option when you are in your second trimester. But, if your condition is manageable through medications or diet, your doctor will likely delay until you've had your baby to undergo the procedure. To avoid gallstones, try taking a low-fat diet that is free of oily and processed foods.

A low amniotic volume is a sign that there isn't sufficient amniotic fluid inside the uterus to help support your growing baby. Every time you see your therapist will examine the size of your uterus and look for signs of the growth. If the caregiver determines that there's only a little or none, they'll schedule an ultrasound test to determine the fluid levels in your body. If they find that it's too low, they'll closely examine your pregnancy to make sure your baby's development is in line with normal by using ultrasounds, biophysical profile as well as non-stress tests. If you're nearing pregnancy or if the baby is not growing well in the womb, your caretaker can either induce you to perform C-sections.

Placenta previa can be discovered early during pregnancy or around that 20th-week ultrasound. The placenta may attach to the wall of your uterus in any direction; it may be posterior or anterior or near the uterus's front or behind the uterus, respectively. Sometimes, however, it may connect in a manner that it completely covers the cervix. This is known as placenta priori. If it completely covers the cervix, then you'll not be permitted to give birth to naturally. Your healthcare provider will have to perform C-section. In reality, most (not the majority) women diagnosed with a placenta previa will are able to undergo an normal birth, due to the fact that the placenta may be removed from the cervix when the baby expands. Your physician will keep an check on your placenta prior to it goes into the labor process at a normal time.

Chapter 13: The Child inside You

What is a baby's appearance at in the Birthing Place?

It is a rapid change for your baby throughout the first trimester as it begins to form in the first stages, particularly towards the beginning the baby does not appear exactly like a baby. But, those tiny cells are hard at work, developing toes, fingers, bones, organs and brain organs.

The first Trimester In the first trimester, it grows to the same size as a seed poppy and all the way to the size of the size of a plum. It's difficult to envision anything getting that big! There are changes happening and hormones are rushing through the body. You might feel nauseated frequently, or you could get sick. The feeling may become less tired than normal. Have a couple of extra naps and take advantage of your extra rest. The sleep you have had will fade into time.

Week 5 is typically what you're at prior to finding out that you're expecting, and the baby has the same size as the size of an apple seed. It is an embryo. it appears similar to the shape of a tadpole. Major organs are beginning to grow along with the digestive, nervous and circulation system. The embryo is very busy!

Week 6: At this point your child is about the dimension of a pea. roughly a quarter inch in length. Face features are beginning to take shape. The heart beats rapidly and blood begins to flow. Fingers and toes have been developed and they are wrapped in webs.

*Week 7: Your tiny one measures about half an inch in length already. Double its size in a week! The brain is on a speedy track, and it is generating around 100 new cells per each minute! The kidneys are working and the little arms and legs start to grow.

*Week 8: The baby is moving around the room although you may not notice it. Webbing is beginning to fall off the toes and fingers, and the tasting buds are developing.

*Week 9: Not just does your infant have the dimensions that of an olive it also has a brand-new name: Fetus! The facial features of her baby are growing fast and, if lucky enough, you could detect the heartbeat during this visit.

"Week 10": your child has grown to be over one inch long. Joints are in motion as her cartilage and bones are developing quickly. Fingernails and hair on her nails are beginning to grow. The girl isn't just moving and kicks, she's also trying to swallow.

Week 11: Your child has grown to over one inch and a half and weighs a quarter of an one ounce. The baby has lost a lot of her look like a tadpole and appears much more like a child. The webbing on her fingers and toes are totally gone.

Week 12: Your child has grown to the size of an apple. It's more than two inches long and almost a half inch in weight. The majority of her systems are completely formed and expanding rapidly. Her reflexes are developing, she's the ability to open and close her fingers and is growing her brain.

The second trimester is when your hormone levels are lowering typically, which results in lesser sickness. You'll notice that the fatigue you've battled over the last 12 weeks decreases and you'll be able to enjoy greater energy. You may even look pregnant now.

"Week 13": The baby is weighing close to 3 inches. The teeth are beginning to grow (below the gum line) as well as her vocal cords are beginning to form. The intestines of her are beginning to move to the right place, and her small fingernails already show fingerprints.

*Week 14: Your infant weighs just one and a half pounds and is more than three inches tall. It's been a busy week for him! You may have already noticed him taking a sip of his thumb. The liver, kidneys, and spleen work hard. Hair that's thin and fuzzy called lanugo is beginning to appear across his entire body.

*Week 15: Your child has increased by an ounce within the space of a week. He measures approximately 4 inches. It's all moving around everywhere; you could be able to feel the motion but it's there. You may even be hearing him experiencing a hiccupping sensation, as every joint and limb are moving.

Week 16: How she's gotten bigger. She's the size of an avocado. She measures little over four and a half inches. She weighs around 3 and 1/2 grams. Hair, including brows and lashes are increasing in size. You can hear her voice.

*Week 17: He's more than five inches tall and 5 ounces heavier. All the cartilage is beginning to change into bone and he's putting on the weight.

Week 18: This infant has the same size as the size of a sweet potato. He has hiccups, yawns is sucks and is able to swallow. The kicks and punches he makes may be be felt in the present. A sound wave at this point could be able to determine his gender.

"Week 19": baby is approximately the size of a mango. It measures six inches in length and carrying a weight of over 8 pounds. The baby is beginning to develop her vernix. This is an oily, white layer which covers the entire body. There will be some when she is born and it's wiped off. It's an anti-skin protectant that assists in keeping her warm inside the baby's womb. The brain of your baby is developing five senses.

Week 20: Your child certainly has grown! She's now getting her taste buds operating. The baby is kicking around like a madman and you might be feeling it for the first time in the week. It's likely that you will receive an ultrasound later this week to assess your baby's health and growth. If it's a good thing or want to find out, the doctor could be able see the gender of the baby if it agrees.

"Week 21": The baby is about ten one and half inches in length currently, and weighs about 12 pounds. The digestive system of her is producing meconium (the initial poop she creates inside her diaper is sticky, black, and tar-like). If she's female, her eggs have already been formed. They are a time supply.

*Week 22: She's getting bigger and taking up plenty of space. It's possible to notice some stretch marks or two at this point If you're thin the belly button could be beginning to show. When you're becoming more discomforted, your girlfriend is snuggling up to rest and it happens in the form of cycles.

Week 23: This is the moment when your "average" baby really starts to fluctuate in terms of size and weight. The baby you have is about 1 foot in length and weighs from 12 to 20 ounces. It's all formed, and is getting heavier. She's watching your heartbeat and to sounds from outside.

Week 24: She's approximately similar to the grapefruit at present. Doctors may recommend to test your glucose levels this week. It is becoming more apparent that you are getting increased movement in your little one. The capillaries she has recently developed have formed and give her a translucent, smooth skin and a more human, organic appearance.

*Week 25: Your infant is now more than an inch long, and she can range from 1 and a half inches to two and one and a half pounds. She is aware of which way is up and what direction is down. She's losing weight, and hair could be growing longer.

Week 26: Her lashes are growing and in the near future she'll be able to look up. The immune system of her is ramping up to cope with life on the outside, and she's beginning to learn how to breathe. The air she breathes isn't there; her lungs are stuffed with amniotic fluid. These practice breathing exercises help her improve her lungs as well as give an opportunity for practice.

Week 27: She's growing weight quickly as well as her lungs growing more powerful. The brain is showing activity, possibly dreaming and thinking. The ultrasounds could show the thumbs sucking. If you're contemplating scheduling a 3D ultrasound scan, now is the right time to book an appointment. Images are improved between weeks 27 and 30.

The third Trimester It's almost there and she's almost there too! There is a possibility that you're more tired because of pain and may you may find yourself waking up frequently in the late at night. If you're unable to sleep and you're tired, try finding something that can help to relax. The breasts already have colonostrum (the feed your baby takes prior to the time when your milk is flowing) and it is possible that you begin to feel Braxton Hicks contractions. They are usually not uncomfortable and can help to tone your part of the uterus that is needed for birth.

"Week 28": The girl is one-quarter of the size of an avocado but can weigh anything from 1 and 1/2 to 2 and 1/2 pounds, and range between thirteen and a quarter inches to just over 14 inches. Her weight is increasing and her skin has lost its youthful look. Her lungs have matured and, if you enter labor, she could make it through in the present. With each passing week her odds increase.

Week 29: Your infant has topped the charts with about 15-16 inches and 2 1/2 to three pounds. You can see him moving around in a flash as his energy levels are high. He's developing white fat deposits. It's possible to notice him wiping.

*Week 30: Your child is now the length of an average cucumber. As his skin becoming smoother, his brain is becoming more curvier. wrinkles are appearing within his brain in order in order to accommodate the brain's development. The young man can now grip with hands, and ultrasounds could demonstrate him holding hands, playing with the umbilical cord!

Week 31 :Your child might now be sixteen inches tall and weigh as much as three and one-half (or greater) pounds. Eye irises are now able to respond to light, and all five senses are all functioning.

*Week 32: She's likely been slouched down in the last week, however don't let it bother you if she's not because there's ample time. It's possible that you both feel as if you're about to run through space.

"Week 33": The child is now weighing between four and five pounds, and is 17 to 18 inches in length. The eyes of your baby are opened while she's awake. Her the sucking and breathing as well as swallowing have become more coordinated. The bones of her are getting also stronger.

Week 34: He's approximately the size of butternut squash. He can recognize and react to your voice, and to your songs. He urinates about 2 cups per each day. Urine is part of amniotic fluid which circulates through the body of your baby every day.

*Week 35: She'll not increase her length in the coming weeks however, she'll keep growing weight. The average gain is one-quarter of a pound every week. If you're pregnant with an infant, the tests will probably be completely gone by now.

*Week 36: In case you aren't yet buying the car seat you want it's the perfect time to buy one. If you own one already, put it in. If the baby was to be born right now it is likely that he will be healthy. If not, the baby may require extra attention at the hospital. If you've not yet prepared a birth schedule it's the perfect moment to create one. The plan should be given an original copy of your birth plan to the caregiver to keep for records, and make certain that they are happy with the birth plan. Baby is gearing for birth and might have turned his head downwards and lowered a little in order to provide you with more breathing space. You may not be seeing him yet. Don't be worried, some babies have to wait until labor begins in order to be placed. The majority of his systems are in good functioning order.

*Week 37 the baby is now full term! The baby is exactly at the size she's supposed to be (but she will increase in weight each week that it is still within the womb). If you experience labor, the family member will never try to hinder you. The baby continues to learn how to breathe and getting ready for the first day of diapers.

*Week 38: A baby can vary from 15 to twenty-two inches tall and weighing in excess of 6 pounds. This will depend on the method you use to develop your baby. Hair may be a quarter of one-inch long (or lesser, a few newborns are born with hair that is full and certain babies come with the fuzz) He's also beginning to lose the vernix.

"Week 39": You child continues to grow in pounds and might grow to larger than a watermelon in the near future. It will be easy to feel as you're in a watermelon as your belly is like a watermelon. You can feel your joints flex while his fingers perhaps dangling over his fingers. Each week, he weighs more and gets smarter, so every week you bring your child in the better equipped he'll be to face all the challenges of life.

*Week 40: If you did get an ultrasound this morning, the weight might differ by more than two pounds. So if your doctor informs you that the baby weighs in at this weight be aware of that. You may go into labor soon, but you may not. First time pregnancies typically runs for 41 weeks and 5 days.

*Weeks 41-43 If you're lucky, you'll have a baby in the past, however should you not have, your doctor could discuss the possibility of induction with you. Your baby is mature and is now living without your womb. Your placenta could become weaker over some time and cause your baby to be lacking nutrients. The majority of babies emerge by themselves after 42nd week. should your caretaker allow you to continue being pregnant for this for a long time, your child will have a healthy birth. It is likely that you are well-prepared for the birth of your baby However, you

might be apprehensive about induction.
very appealing.

Can You Reduce Birth Defects?

The causes for many kinds of birth defects are not known however, there are a few actions you can take to attempt to avoid some.

See your physician for regularly scheduled prenatal visits.

Make a pre-conception appointment in order to see if as well as your father are susceptible to certain genetic conditions.

Make sure you take enough folic acid prior to and throughout the pregnancy period to avoid neural tube problems such as spina bifida.

• Stop drinking, smoking or smoking cigarettes and. They are all linked to birth defects.

Check with your doctor regarding the medications you're using. Certain drugs have been reported to be a cause of birth defects.

Check that your vaccinations are up-to-date prior to getting pregnant.

Avoid harmful substances such as paint thinners and pesticides lead-based paints and polluted water to mention some.

Although these measures won't be able to prevent the birth defect in all cases however, they're positive steps to take in the right direction.

Caution: What You Take May Harm Your Baby

When we think of the things that may affect their infant They usually consider smoking cigarettes, street drugs or even alcohol. A lot of people don't realize that the medicines they're given by their doctor can harm their child. This is the reason it's essential to consult your physician about the medications you are taking prior to conception or at the time you begin to think about having children. Some antidepressants haven't been studied on women who are pregnant however they have been proven to induce birth defects in rats.

There are times when doctors do not realize the impact of drugs on the fetus until it's for them to know, therefore check if there's an alternative to the drug or if you're able to go without taking the medication for 9 months.

The most common medications to stay clear of during pregnancy include things such like naproxen, ibuprofen and aspirin. Ibuprofen is the principal ingredient in Advil as well as Motrin as well as naproxen that is the principal ingredient in Aleve can reduce circulation of blood to the newborn. Aspirin thins blood vessels and may cause bleeding issues in both. If you suffer from indigestion, do not take Pepto-Bismol. Instead, consult your physician about other options. If you suffer from an infection, you should avoid using all products that contain Guaifenesin. It can raise the chance of developing neural tube defects. This can be found in many products such as Mucinex as well as Robitussin. It is crucial to inform your physician about any medication you're on, be it prescription or other.

Some teas could have negative effects on your pregnancies. Green teas can contain caffeine, and it crosses the placenta. A few herbal teas may be hazardous too. Be sure to talk with your healthcare provider regarding any issues you may have.

How can you ensure a healthy brain development of your baby in the First Trimester

The most effective way to make sure the brain of your baby is well and remains healthy is to stay clear of any medication that can lead to neural tube defects quit drinking, smoking or taking any street drug and also through taking folic acids. It is also possible to encourage your the brain of your baby to grow stronger through healthy eating and by taking the fish oil (DHA) supplements. Stress reduction can help in this regard.

Why Do Babies Kick Inside the Womb?

The phrase "kicking" doesn't really cover what babies do during the birth. The baby moves his arms and legs, stretches his legs, turns his head and bends legs and arms. This helps prepare him for what's to come on the outside. Take a look at the moves people perform in order to build their muscles. You bend your knees, move their torsos around, raise the arms, and lower them. This is exactly what babies are doing. This is just the first step towards a fit robust baby.

The first signs of movement can be felt at around four or five weeks of age, but you will not be able detect it till later. Baby is small and is too deep inside your stomach for you to be able to feel it. Certain women feel movements from as little at 13 weeks. However, some don't experience any sensation until they reach 25 weeks. Being able to feel your that your baby moves in the first time often referred to as a quickening which is considered to be one of the best emotions a woman during pregnancy experiences. Every move is a sign that you're making a difference in the world.

Chapter 14: Pre-Delivery What You Need to Know?

Why Would a Childbirth Class Be Helpful?

The classes for children can inform you on the impending birth as well as teach relaxation techniques and provide important information on what kinds of pain relief options are offered in your hospital. The type of course you choose to take will depend on the kind of birth you wish to experience. If you're having your baby at an in-hospital facility, you'll probably end up having some form of pain relief. Childbirth classes provide the understanding necessary to pick the most appropriate option for you. If you're hoping to have natural birth that can be a non-medicated birth but it's important to be aware of your choices if you experience a tense situation. Many women choose medications to ease pain, but they do not know the potential adverse effects that this substance could cause on themselves as well as the child. A babybirth class will help you identify the side effects you're likely to be exposed to in the event that pain becomes severe. But, there are various types of childbirth classes that are available, at the hospital as well as outside of your pocket.

What Types of Childbirth Classes Are There?

Certain insurances cover childbirth classes in your physician's clinic or the hospital. If you do not want to pay a significant costs out of your pocket, this might be the most suitable option to start. Learn about the classes your institution has to offer and if your insurance covers the cost of classes. If you're able to cover out-of-pocket expenses However, you are able to be pickier. If you are looking for a class be sure to determine if it is compatible with the expectations you have for its execution. If the class is in person course (versus the self-study or online option) learn about the instructor's qualifications or experiences is, as well as how many couples will join the class the instructor. It is also important to consider the location of the class. evaluation, and so is the times the classes are scheduled to take place. It's probably not any good to book the class for childbirth that's 30 minutes from you and begins at ten minutes late after working.

Classes in Lamaze: Lamaze classes aren't just about teaching you breathing techniques and relaxation methods however, they also instruct the basics of normal births as well as breastfeeding, medication C-sections, as well as the basics of labor. A majority of Lamaze classes last minimum 12 hours in duration. See   www.lamazeinternational.org   for more information regarding Lamaze Childbirth classes.

It is the Bradley Method or American Academy of Husband Coached Childbirth: The Bradley Method teaches childbirth as naturally occurring human activity. They will teach the techniques for natural birth and provide you with the skills of how to advocate for yourself. Bradley Method Bradley Method emphasizes relaxation and natural birth. The course lasts about 12 weeks to complete. So don't be too late to book the classes. For more information on the Bradley Method, visit their website at www.bradleybirth.com.

International Childbirth Education Association: Instructors that are trained by ICEA they are typically educational courses offered by hospitals and doctors office. They will teach you labor techniques and comfort techniques, along with medications as well as possible issues. For more information about ICEA class on childbirth or find the nearest instructor go to www.icea.org.

Hypnobabies, a course that is available either in person or a self-study at home course. It's usually out of pocket and the self-study kits is available on their website, or on Amazon.com. This course is intended for natural births that are not medicated it can be utilized in the privacy of your home, at an birthing centre, or in a hospital. The class teaches you about the way your body functions during birth, labor as well as after. The program teaches you what to pay attention to the process of labor, with an overall aim of assisting you to have an uninvolved, pain-free and drug-free peaceful birth experience. Find out more details about the program at www.hypnobabies.com. There exist other classes in self-hypnosis for birth on the market, but this takes a deeper examination of the body. It also provides you with techniques will be useful all through your pregnancy and afterward. This class is especially beneficial when you're determined to have an unmedicated birth.

There are a variety of classes for children, but none of them has been discussed here. Which classes are offered to your area has a lot in common with what's offered in your region. Discover what classes the local hospitals offer as well as what's being offered in your local area.

What are the reasons you should avoid unneeded medical interventions First What are unneeded medical procedures? The exact definition of these interventions may vary depending on the individual. In my case, for instance, I consider monitors for fetal growth, Pitocin, and IVs as unnecessary in the event of childbirth. The medical profession, as well as hospitals believe that childbirth is as if it were a condition and treat it accordingly. It is monitored closely. There are some areas where you aren't allowed to eat drinks or food while you are in labour. It is recommended to have an IV that contains saline to help you stay hydrated. It is mandatory to stay stationary, mostly in a reclined position, and you aren't allowed to move or rock at times. The birth process doesn't have to be painful but in conjunction with these procedures the result is often. If you don't have water or food the body rapidly runs out of fuel. With no assistance from gravity, some infants struggle to descend. If they aren't able to get towards a position that is more comfortable in order to reduce pain, the discomfort can get unbearably intense. This can lead to the use of pain medication and can have the effect of lowering blood pressure as well as slowing the rate of labor. Certain medications can have negative effects on individuals, and many patients who take them notice they are shaking out of control nauseating or vomiting. The drugs may also contribute to pitocin-induced contractions that do not occur naturally and can cause among those that are the most uncomfortable. Most often, pain medication have side effects that can cause C-sections, forceps, suction or force-pushing prior to when mom's body is prepared to push.

Another treatment which is not needed in the majority of situations is the artificial rupturing of membranes (AROM). This is an approach used by doctors to help get labor moving faster. The doctor inserts a stick-like instrument that has a small hook on the other end of it into the vagina, and then up into the Cervix. Then they hook it over your membranes, and then pull. The water will be broken, which will increase contractions and strengthen them. This makes your baby and you in a time-line. After the waters have been broken, doctors typically allow you 12 hours for the birth of your baby. If they think you're not working fast enough, or if your labor has stopped and they are unable to help, they may prescribe Pitocin to help speed up the progress of your labor. Numerous issues can be attributed to AROM. If your water supply is damaged and leaking, it becomes easier to allow bacteria to your urinary tract. This is the reason you're placed on a routine. You are scared of getting sick which can be harmful to you as well as your baby. What they've achieved by performing AROM is that they've removed the cushion, which helps take the shock of contractions. If the labor isn't moving quickly enough, they'll provide you with Pitocin. This can make contractions are stronger and could cause you to opt to utilize drugs and/or an epidural.

The epidural should reduce pain from the lower part of your waist to. An anesthesiologist inserts the needle between your vertebrae to insert it into the spinal cord. When the muscles contract, and you are asked to lie on your feet and lie down over your stomach, while they attempt to introduce the needle. This can be uncomfortable when you are contracting at all. A catheter is put over the needle, and then through the hole in the spinal column. This will inject a medication into the spinal column that blocks the pain that comes from the puncture all right down to your feet. The majority of the drugs are within this mix and often you're given the option of pushing a button at least every 15 minutes to give doses according to the need. There are two kinds of epidurals available, the standard epidural as well as one called the "walking" epidural, though this latter one is an error, since it is not permitted to go anywhere after the epidural is placed. There are some side effects associated with every drug, and epidurals are no one of them. One of the most commonly reported adverse effects is a rise of blood pressure. Another one is a slowing of labor. The majority of women are instructed to push once they're 10 centimeters dilate in the case of an epidural, it is common that you aren't able to figure out the best way to push. It can take for several hours. If it continues for over a long period, the physician might decide to do C-section or utilize suction or forceps.

Another medical treatment which is a bit out of date is the episiotomy. A majority of physicians do not carry out episiotomies. However, some perform them. Episiotomy refers to a process that allows the doctor to cut your peritoneum prior to delivery of the head of your baby. It is a cut which runs from the lower part in your vagina's opening to the anus. The cut is painful and can take longer to heal than the tear. Also, it is more painful than tears. It was the case that medical professionals believed that a more clean cut was the better option as it was more easy to clean up and sew. But, if you choose the natural fiber of a plant and cut it into pieces, you'll notice the ease with which the ends join. If you dampen it just slightly, it appears as if it's brand new. Take the same fibre and slice it into one straight line by using cutters. Are the ends joined easier? They do not, and will be unable to stick when wet. The skin is the same. The simple tear heals better than cuts. But, in some instances an episiotomy may make the difference between breaking the vagina, or getting a clean cut. It shouldn't be done randomly.

Unfortunately, these procedures have been frequently used in hospitals setting that the majority of medical professionals and nurses haven't witnessed an unmedicated, natural birth during their entire career. The medical procedures are a result of a waterfall. After you receive the IV, getting medications for pain becomes simpler. Also, it is simpler for doctors to prescribe Pitocin. When Pitocin is present there is mandatory to take the painkiller, even though a very few women have managed to overcome the pitocin-triggered contractions without using medications. Pitocin may over stimulate the uterus, causing discomfort in the infant. It is not possible to move around when you're taking Pitocin as you'll be required to monitor your fetus continuously often. Many occasions, movements could make the monitor slip or "lose" the baby's heartbeat and scare the nursing team. When you're in a position and cannot move, your contractions will be more uncomfortable.

If your labor lasts for a long time, and you're thirsty, exhausted and thirsty, it's easy to seek out medications. Medicines can cause side effects that may affect both you and the child. That's why classes for childbirth are crucial. If you're looking for a safe pregnancy that yields a healthy outcome it's crucial to be aware of how the common medication used in the birth process and consider whether you'd like to put your life at risk on your baby and yourself. If you're able get a safe, natural birth, it's due to your decision to avoid numerous unnecessary medical procedures.

Chapter 15: What Happens During Pregnancy?

The experience of being pregnant is something completely different. It's both the most amazing experience of an entirely new phase of life as well as a painfully discomforting (and often difficult) event all in the same. It's a rollercoaster of physical and emotional highs as well as lows. Both result from the body and brain getting flooded with different hormones (or the hormones you're used to consuming being reduced). Contrary to what you may think it is considered to be a clinical process as the state in which the embryo, or fetus, expands and grows in the womb of the mother and in which the child to be born depends on its mother for the survival of. The pregnancy is split into three stages, which are comprised of three months. This totals nine months of gestation. Mother's body goes through many adjustments to help accommodate the expanding baby and to support its growth and growth.

To support and accommodate the baby's growing in the womb, our bodies begin to release or reduce certain hormones throughout the pregnancy. These hormones mostly affect the reproductive organs of the mother, however some are systemic too. As an example, a hormone known as relaxin is released during pregnancy, which causes joints to stretch more. This allows for stretch in the pelvic region in order to support the baby's growing body however, it also makes every other joint more adaptable. A lot of pregnant women notice that they're able to extend more than they ever have previously during their pregnancy and this leads to amazing form using various yoga postures!

The cardiovascular system takes an immense amount of stress because of pregnancy. This is because in the course of pregnancy, the heart pumps out more blood, and it does so at a higher pace. After all, the heart has to support two people currently, and not just one. This is essential for blood to efficiently circulate and also provide adequate oxygen and nutrients for the growing fetus.

There is good and negative, but. Blood pressure issues can arise in this increased stress of the cardio-vascular system. It is easier for blood flow to be concentrated in the uterus as the developing baby requires increased oxygen and nutrition. The result is that the organs and brain are receiving lesser blood flow than they did prior to pregnancy. It can cause nausea or dizziness. Other changes expectant mothers may encounter at different stages of her pregnancy.

The first sign of pregnancy is typically following a missed menstrual cycle. Signs of pregnancy are nausea, vomiting tenderness of the breasts frequent urination, being fatigued easily. One of the best methods to determine the if you're pregnant is to look for what's called"BFP" or "BFP"--a large fat positive! BFP is a BFP is the result of a pregnancy test that is positive with a pregnancy test at home. When pregnant the vagina and cervix occasionally turn blue because of an increase in blood flow into the area (this is known as Chadwick's Sign). "Goodell's sign" is that refers to the weakening of the vagina during pregnancy. Hegar's sign is a reference to variations in the structure of a uterus that is pregnant. These are all signs of the possibility of pregnancy. There are two reliable methods to determine if you are experiencing a pregnancy. One is using the use of a Doppler device, where the microphone is placed on the abdomen of the woman for the purpose of detecting audible infant heart sounds as well as the visualisation of the outline of the fetus using ultrasound technology. Heart sounds from the fetus may not be heard until 12 weeks of pregnancy however ultrasound technology makes it possible to determine if a baby is pregnant in as early as six weeks into gestation in the time that the embryo is less than the size of a grain rice!

After confirmation of your pregnancy when you are confirmed to be pregnant, you will begin experiencing more changes happen in your body when your baby expands. The first third trimester (first 3 months) your body may exhibit little external physical change. The abdomen only increases slightly. The baby bump doesn't have noticeable in the majority of cases with the exception of some multiparous women, i.e. those who've had an entire term pregnancy prior to. In the first trimester the uterus is usually only barely above the pubic bone at or near the level of pelvic vertebrae. The fertilized egg is rapidly divided and forms the embryo. The embryo is later (around two months after the gestation) is referred to as the Fetus.

The trimester that begins in the first trimester is a phase of the development of the embryo as well as organogenesis in the infant. Organs of the baby start forming, starting by the heart. Faces also begin to form, including the eyes. Blood cells start to form and circulate in the embryo. Placentas are also created in this period, which can provide food for your infant through the whole gestational period through the course of your pregnancy.

In the second trimester the uterus expands in size rapidly. The uterus expands in order to fit to accommodate the growing baby. The size of the uterus begins to increase beyond the pelvic bones to the umbilicus. This causes the baby's stomach to grow larger. At the conclusion of the second trimester, mother could begin feeling the movements of her fetus. While the mother is lying down, she can be able to feel her newborn "kick" inside her womb. Uterine contractions, also known as Braxton-Hicks contractions, may be evident around the same time. This isn't a sign of premature or unplanned birth, unless contractions are frequent and regular and trigger bleeding or pain. Sometimes, the expecting mother could feel exhausted or experience trouble breathing in deeply. It is because of the increasing uterus pushing upward pressure on the expecting mother's diaphragm.

At the end of the third trimester the uterus has become large. It is now an extent that has significant impacts on the organs around it. Mothers' posture begins with a lordotic "sway-backed" posture, where abdominal muscles extend outwards and the curvature of her lower back gets more over-exaggerated. The term "sway-back" is used to describe"the "pride of pregnancy." The pace of breathing is increased as the baby grows, leaving moms feeling exhausted and out exhausted more often. A growing uterus places pressure on the diaphragm, causing an increase in the rate of breathing. This also places pressure on the bladder of urine, which causes moms to have frequently trips to the toilet. Rectums also take pressure of the uterus, sometimes causing constipation as the pregnancy progresses. Urinary contractions rise in frequency, and then become more frequent and consistent when the date for the birth approaches. The cervix shrinks in the process of softening, and then becoming more flexible. The breasts begin to expand and become full of colonostrum as they prepare to breastfeed upon birth.

The infant already has all organs within the body. The last one to grow are the lung. All of these are ways in that the mother's body is preparing for the upcoming delivery of her child, as well all of the baby's organs prepare themselves to transition into life beyond the womb. Between 37 and 42 weeks of gestation it is believed that the baby is "full term" and ready to be with its parents and the world.

Chapter 16: Discomforts of Pregnancy

Growing a baby in your body can be thrilling and inspiring. It can, however, be among the most challenging times in the life of a woman. The body can be subject to stress in all ways that are emotional, physical as well as mental. Physically, the body experiences radical and swift changes as the pregnancy develops in each new trimester. The fetus is growing quickly and is able to absorb blood nutrients from the mother's body through the placenta. Mother's body also makes hormones which make its components, particularly the uterus capable to support the growing fetus.

The first trimester

At the beginning of your first trimester the breasts may feel uncomfortable or even painful as they start to seem heavier than they normally do. It is possible to become uneasy, especially at the beginning of the day. It is also possible to experience nausea. Vomiting and nausea can trigger lots of discomfort in the beginning of your trimester. This can even reduce the nutrition available to the developing female fetus. Also, there is an increased sensitization to specific flavors and smells. The scent of bread baking can create a gush in your mouth, as well as when you meet the craving for food, it could be the most delicious food you've ever eaten! But the drawback to an increased sense of scent is that the smell of garbage when garbage day comes around can have your stomach doing dance.

Nausea and vomiting is reactions of the body to hormone changes that take place in the pregnancy. The symptoms can be brought on due to low blood pressure or blood sugar levels, emotional stress, eating too much fat, or the overuse of spices on the menu and the low level of iron and vitamin B6 within the body. Vomiting and nausea usually start gradually diminishing by the middle of the first trimester. If nausea and vomiting continue through the fifth month of pregnancy, it could be that you suffer from a condition known as hyperemesis gravidarum. It is possible that the vomiting and nausea possibly be an indicator of other, more serious issues. Check with your obstetrician in the event that it happens to you.

There is a chance that you are exhausted and sleepy all throughout the day. Many women might be prone to fainting or dizziness. It is possible that you are making more frequent trips to the toilet. The changes in progesterone and estrogen levels can also impact the mucus linings in the body. This is the reason why most pregnant women get up with a nasal congestion. Avoid colds or allergy medications, however it is most likely due to hormones and is it is not caused by viruses or a bacteria (not forgetting the warnings when taking these kinds of medications during pregnancy!). It's good to know that they aren't indicators that your health or body are in danger. These indications are only that your body is adapting to the arrival and development of your baby. The majority of discomforts in the first and second trimesters can be a result of responses of your body's response to fluctuations in hormone levels.

The second trimester

The majority of first symptoms of the first trimester will diminish by the end of the second quarter of the year, because the body becomes used to the idea of being pregnant. After the second trimester, you'll notice that the "baby bump" will start showing. Breathing gets a little more difficult due to the expanding uterus pushing the diaphragm up, which compresses the lung tissue. Defecation can also begin to be challenging. It could be because of the hormonal effects and Vitamins you're taking for pregnancy as well as the stress of your uterus during the your bowel movements. Or it could be a combination of the three!

Acid reflux and hyperacidity (heartburn) may be because of the hormonal changes that a woman who is pregnant encounters. The lower esophageal muscle (between the stomach and the esophagus) could weaken, which allows the stomach acid to flow to the stomach and into the esophagus. This can cause the downward pressure exerted by the uterus against the stomach. Foods can be unpalatable because of the heartburn.

The changes in skin appear to be more obvious. The skin can darken and then become more rough. The face may be swollen and freckle-like also known as chloasma be visible. Within the abdomen there is a dark line that runs between the umbilicus and the pubis can start to appear. It is referred to as linea in nigra (from the Latin meaning "black line").

The third trimester

In the third trimester the baby is expected to grow in stature, and begin to exert stress on the organs adjacent to it. The uterus will expand upward and outwards as the diaphragm moves upwards, the lungs are constrained and breathing will require a great deal more effort. The uterus presses against the bladder to increase the frequency of urine. Constipation could become worse when the bowel gets pressurized by the Uterus.

Hemorrhoids may begin to develop when the bowels of the lower part continue to be compressed due to the contraction of the uterus. They are a result of the wall of the intestine, usually located in the anal and rectal area. They can trigger defecation that could be uncomfortable and the rectum can even be bleeding if the hemorrhoids create anal fissures.

The leg cramps can become worse by 3rd trimester. The mother-to-be will frequently wake during the night with leg cramps. The reason for this is shifts in circulation of blood and the reduction in blood calcium levels. The infant requires more calcium in the third trimester when the muscles and bones grow and begin to develop. The levels of blood calcium in the mother decrease as calcium gets diverted to the child.

When the abdomen (and the child inside) grows and expand, lots of stress is put on the back of the lower part. The most frequent backaches occur in the third trimester after the baby has become substantially bigger. Varicose veins can also begin appearing. They may also look enlarged and swelling. Breasts begin to get full of colostrum due to hormones known as prolactin as well as oxytocin. Apart from helping with lactation, oxytocin is also a trigger for contractions in the uterus. These contractions are more frequent and consistent when you are closer to your due date for due date.

Chapter 17: Natural Remedies for Pregnancy Complaints

The hormonal and physical changes to the body that occur during pregnancy can reduce the amount of joy and joy initially felt by mothers-to-be. There are many remedies available to treat the discomforts, unintentional negative effects could affect the mother as well as the child. It's better and more secure to seek out natural remedies whenever feasible. Below are some methods to deal with these issues in a natural and effective way to ensure an enjoyable, healthy, and relaxed pregnancy.

Nausea

Nausea is regarded as the top complaint among expecting mothers. Popularity in the pregnancy period has grown to stereotypical levels The queasy mother-to be is an integral part of the media, ranging from sitcom shows to comedy blogs.

Nausea is typically caused by abrupt changes in the hormones of a pregnant woman. In the early stages of the pregnancy period, hormonal changes can be something your body is not used to and can cause a lot of stress. However, there is a silver lining for this, however. The nausea, although sometimes extreme and extremely painful for some moms, typically (thankfully!) disappears towards the end the 1st trimester. It is not a requirement for medication. If it continues over the course of three months or gets more severe seek out your obstetrician because it could require medical intervention. If not, it may be necessary just a couple of minor adjustments in the area of exercise and diet.

Nausea could also be caused due to low blood sugar levels, particularly in the mornings, after breakfast is eaten. An energy-rich snack (such as a piece turkey or jerky) prior to bed could aid. In the event that nausea triggers nausea following the intake of prenatal vitamins early in the day take them before going to the bedtime to determine whether they can be kept down. In the end, nutrition is crucial as prenatal vitamins provide vital to improve nutrition for the mother-to-be as well as her child growing. If you wake up in the morning, take a slow rise off the bed, rather than leaping up to get on your feet. Sometimes being too quick can cause people feel nauseated and dizzy So being cautious in your initial steps throughout the day could prove beneficial. Consume dried peach leaves anise, red raspberry Fennel seed, ginger teas (or perhaps simply ginger ale, in the event that you enjoy infrequently carbonated drinks) to reduce nausea during the day. Warm water with a teaspoon cider vinegar could also aid. Ground ginger could also give relief either through making the root inspirable or inhaling it. Incorporate foods high in iron to your food plan (but be aware that iron can cause constipation so ensure to drink enough water). A lot of women swear by drinking soda crackers before breakfast while some women discover an increase in regularity of meals and reducing the amount of food consumed (eating less food but eating it more often) helps keep vomiting under control.

Aromatherapy oils contain fragrances of chamomile, rose and lavender for massage. Inhaling smoke or smoke from aromatherapy oils isn't advised for women suffering from chronic respiratory illnesses, because asthma symptoms can be brought on or become worse. (Note that it is advised to avoid burning aromatic candles or essential oils for the first three months of pregnancy.)

Mothers who are bleeding are advised to be careful when using ginger. Patients with bleeding disorders or those using anticoagulants must check with their physician prior to making plans to consume ginger. The herb also slows down blood clotting as well as increasing the risk of bleeding that is excessive.

Heartburn

It is known as heartburn. (or acid reflux) is a very stressful experience during pregnancy, particularly when eating food. The severity of heartburn can increase during pregnancy, due to the growth of the baby pushing the uterus upwards to the stomach. This causes acid to flow through the stomach to the esophagus. This causes acid reflux. Make sure to stand standing up for one hour following eating since lying down can make the acids rise through the esophagus that causes heartburn to become more severe. Make sure that your meals are small and eat it at regular times throughout your entire day. Milk or yogurt can reduce the acidity in the stomach Therefore, these dairy foods can be a good snack option. Do not eat high-fat food items or foods with a lot of spice. Drinking a glass of warm milk and a teaspoon of honey may help ease heartburn discomfort.

Lactose-intolerant mothers need to talk with their doctor. It is possible that they will need to take lactase (enzyme to break down lactose from milk) or opt for lactose-free milk as well as dairy substitutes.

The fainting and dizziness can be a cause.

In pregnancy, blood may accumulate in your lower body, reducing oxygen and blood flow to the brain. The common occurrence of fainting and dizziness consequences of this type of situation. Be sure to avoid prolonged periods of sitting when you can. Increase venous return and blood flow by stretching and relaxing your legs and butt muscles during the day. If you are lying down, you should lie on your left side (and be sure to avoid lying on your stomach following the beginning of your first trimester because it puts pressure on large blood vessels that may reduce blood flow to your body and the expanding foetus). Adjust your body's position gradually (from sitting to standing or reverse). When you start to feel like you're about to faint then sit down and take a rest. Inhale slowly and deeply to increase oxygen levels. If you are experiencing heat take the necessary steps to remain cool. Temperatures that are hot can increase your dizziness and can result in fainting make sure you find areas with air conditioning to unwind in whenever possible. If you don't have access to a cooling system, you can take refreshing baths or showers, and put a cool, moist cloth on your forehead or wrapped over your neck to stop you from rising.

Leg cramps

An effective way to keep against leg cramps is by increasing the amount of calcium you consume. These cramps usually result from lower levels of calcium. Women's bodies require high levels of calcium especially during pregnancy because it is crucial in the growth of the foetus. Calcium-rich dairy products such as milk and cheese. Yogurt can also be a great sources of calcium. Certain leafy vegetables are filled with calcium. These include mustard greens, kale, and mustard. If you notice a cramp in your calves and you are unable to move your feet towards the body. Stay there until the pain diminishes.

If you suffer from an ongoing condition or are using other medications, talk to your doctor prior to adding the amount of calcium you consume. The drugs that are cardiovascular, like are more potent in the presence of excessive levels of calcium. Patients who have a tendency to develop kidney stones ought to be cautious about the increase in calcium via dietary supplementation or supplements since kidney stones can get worse with high levels of calcium.

Backaches

The back pain of pregnant women usually stems from the extra burden of an expanding abdomen. The relief it brings can be achieved by receiving an excellent back massage. The pelvic rocking exercise can increase the flexibility and strength of the back muscles in the lower part and also. If you are sleeping, make use of small pillows to help support your spine and legs. Lay on your back using a pillow between your knees in order to ensure that your spine and pelvis are in a proper alignment during sleeping. Shoes with high heels that are flat or which provides stability and support. Also, consider the orthotic insoles that are designed to assist the arch of the feet. Engage in stretching routines every day. Hatha yoga is an excellent option for expecting mothers. Warm or heated compresses is beneficial in the case of compresses being placed on the muscles that are aching for a couple of minutes.

The pain can also be caused by overstretching from bad body mechanics and poor posture. Utilize proper lifting practices. Use knee bends for lifting anything regardless of how lightweight or heavy it might be. The water can reduce tension on the spine, which makes it an excellent mode of exercise moderate for expecting mothers. Herbal supplements can also help ease back pain during pregnancy. A infusion of St. John's wort can be consumed orally by adding fifteen to 25 drops in the warm water in a glass and then drinking it each few hours. If you've got an allergy history don't take St. John's wort, because it may cause allergic reactions in sensitive people. Some preparations also include alcohol, and are not advised for women who are pregnant. Talk to your doctor about alternatives or suggestions for safer versions that contain St. John's wort.

Pelvic Pain

The infant's weight causes stress on the pelvis which causes discomfort. The expansion that occurs gradually of the pelvic inlet during pre-birth preparation can create painful pelvic pain. It is important to keep exercising frequently, and get sufficient pelvic rest throughout your whole day. Like back pain, occasionally applying warm, scaly compresses on the affected area may provide some relief. Yoga poses are that is known as "cat and cow pose" in which you sit on your fours on the floor, and lower your stomach towards the ground, while arching your back (and afterwards, you can round your back to the reverse and make the "C" shape with your spine while crouching) which can prove beneficial in relieving pelvic pain for pregnant women as well as being a fantastic stretching of the spine!

Colds, coughs, and colds

An irritable nose during the morning can be very typical during pregnancy. It can be due to hormonal changes you're going through. However, it doesn't necessarily suggest you're suffering from the flu. But, a pregnant woman has a higher risk of contracting colds and coughs as compared to women who do not. A runny nose and coughing signify that you're suffering from the flu. Do not take over-the-counter medicines for colds since some may seriously harm the baby's nervous system and organ growth.

Enhance your immune system and keep you from recurring infections. Consume a balanced diet and boost your intake of zinc and vitamin C. Vitamin B-complex can also assist in boosting your immune system in times of stress. If you are suffering from sinus infection, take a bite of garlic or onion during your meal, since the wonderful aroma of these bulbs has antibacterial capabilities.

Aromatherapy using eucalyptus and lemon, tea tree as well as lavender, can be beneficial. Put 2 drops of each of these oils into a bowl filled with warm water, then breathe in the steam for around 10 minutes, or until the water becomes cold. Check with your physician before taking this if you suffer from allergies, or have chronic respiratory conditions like asthma. You can add a few drops lemon in your usual drink or warm water for faster recovery from colds. Lemon is full of vitamin C. vitamin C can boost your immune system unlike anything other (and aside from that, the water of citrus tastes tasty!).

Constipation

Changes in hormones and pressure exerted by the uterus could result in constipation. The uterus can compress the bowels and slows down peristalsis. To prevent constipation, you should eat the foods which are high in fiber. Whole grain food items have a lot of levels of fiber, so if you're fan of white bread, here's an unpleasant news for you that it's time to change to nine-grain. The fruits and vegetables are excellent sources of fiber particularly when consumed raw. So, try to have a salad once a each day throughout your pregnancy in order in order to reduce constipation. Iron supplements in the prenatal vitamins may result in constipation. Therefore, make sure you drink more fluids during pregnancy, particularly water (yes that's even though you have to make frequent trips to the toilet). Take a drink of prune juice whenever you need to ease the constipation. Talk to your physician before drinking prune juice if are also taking other medicines in case it causes negative interactions. When you experience the urge to for a bowel movement, go to the bathroom. Avoid putting it into since this may make constipation worsen, and could lead to more problems, like hemorrhoids. Do not strain your bowels when moving them. Training helps to improve peristalsis and stop constipation.

Hemorrhoids

Hemorrhoids are weakening parts of the intestinal wall. They are usually associated with constipation. Be careful not to strain while you defecate so as to decrease the strain on the walls of your intestines. The gravid uterus already creating pressure constant on the intestinal tract, and straining when excreting waste can create more pressure, which makes hemorrhoids more likely happen. They can be painful and even begin to bleed. Use baking soda to treat the hemorrhoids that are exposed or add it to the water in your bath. The juice of lemon or witch hazel are also a great option for cleansing the area to lessen the swelling. Make sure to use witch hazel in moderation but be aware that it could trigger an allergic reaction in certain people. The sitz baths made of herbal ingredients can help reduce itching and swelling caused by hemorrhoids. Similar to all herbal remedies take care when adding herbs to your sitz baths since allergies can be present in people who are susceptible.

High blood pressure

An increase in blood pressure could result from anxiety and stress, or may be an actual physiological reaction to hormones. Medical treatments are not usually advised for women who are pregnant. It is important to keep your blood pressure within a reasonable range since high blood pressure could cause preeclampsia or the condition known as eclampsia (which is defined as life-threatening elevated blood pressure as well as convulsions). Be assured, however. It is possible to lower your blood pressure by using natural ways.

Regular exercise keeps the heart healthy. Swimming and walking are excellent options for exercising during pregnancy and also easy yoga. Take a healthy and balanced diet that includes fresher fruits and vegetables (remember you've heard of the "salad a day" from earlier?). Cucumbers, in particular, are excellent to lower blood pressure. Reduce the risk of high blood pressure and Eclampsia with adequate quantities of protein. Limit intake of red meat. Choose protein sources that are healthier such as turkey, chicken as well as non-predatory fish, and also green vegetables.

If you are a smoker, stop immediately! Smoking cigarettes can have a devastating effect for you as well as your growing infant, such as the rise in blood pressure and the slowed growth of your fetus and the development of the baby. If you stop smoking, it can lead to the reduction of blood pressure by several points within a matter of hours from the time you quit smoking your last smoking session. It is the most crucial option you have for your own health and your baby's health.

It is likely that you have heard salt is one of the main culprits for elevated blood pressure. Don't completely eliminate salt out of your daily diet. All women require sodium for survival! If you are consuming too much salt and you are frequenting the salt shaker frequently than you would like, attempt to decrease your intake of salt. Cut down or eliminate caffeine such as the cola and coffee. Nettles, lime flowers, dandelions, or even raspberries leaf teas can be good alternative. Juice of half the lemon or lime and a half cup of water, plus 2 teaspoons of tartar cream can be consumed once per day. Repeat after two days. The process may lower the blood pressure. But, if you're suffering from an ongoing condition, you should consult your physician prior to trying the herbal treatment, since medicines you're currently having may cause negative interactions with the herbs. Try to avoid stressful situations as much as you can. Be positive in your surroundings.

Preeclampsia

Preeclampsia can be described by consistently excessively high blood pressure. It can cause an eclampsia (leading to potentially dangerous seizures) when left untreated. If you are suffering from hypertension, consume ample amounts of bananas as well as lightly cooked peels of potatoes. These are foods rich in potassium that could help stop eclampsia, or seizures. The total daily calories consumed must be 2400 or more calories in the pregnancy. Drinking beet juice raw, about four ounces a day will help to balance the ratio of sodium and potassium (or "electrolyte balance"). You can take a vitamin B-complex supplement to help reenergize your kidneys and improves blood pressure control. It is possible to drink tea made of young dandelion leafs, because they are rich in calcium and potassium, and can help reduce the appearance of edema, which is causing many pregnancy-related discomfort birds at once. If you're suffering from a heart problem and take cardiovascular medications it is possible to stay clear of dandelion leaf. Calcium and potassium enhance the effectiveness of these medications and trigger negative reactions. Calcium and potassium could also cause a worsening of cardiovascular disease It is recommended to talk with your physician first in case you suffer from one or more of them before starting any regimen of herbal remedies.